# SleepWell:

# Surgery and Obstetrics & Gynecology

Vol. 2

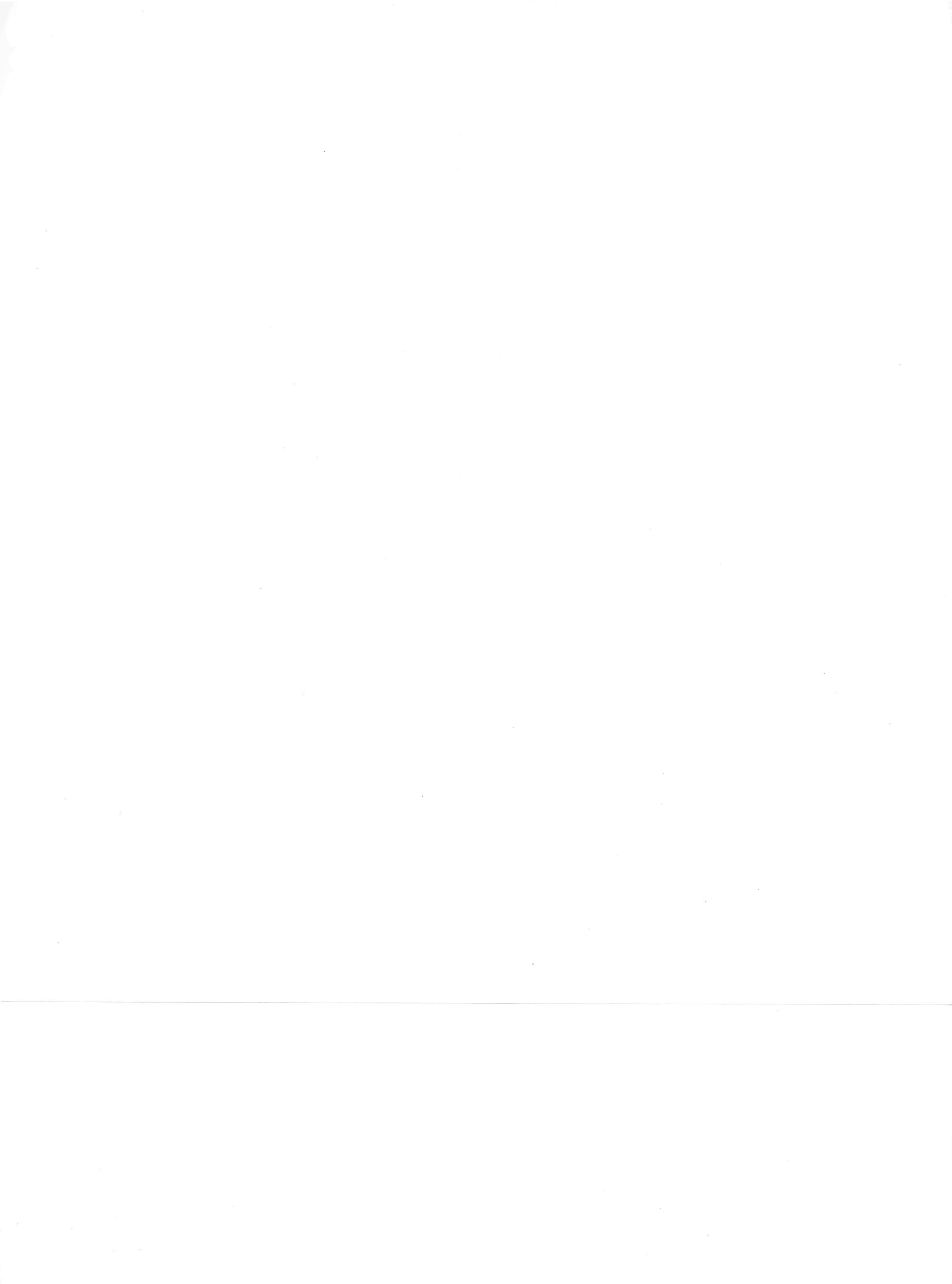

# SleepWell: Surgery and Obstetrics & Gynecology

Vol. 2

**Edited by:**

***E. Douglas Norcross, MD***
Associate Professor of Surgery
Medical University of South Carolina
Attending Surgeon
Medical University Hospital
Charleston, South Carolina

***Paige R. Gernt, MD***
Assistant Professor of Obstetrics and Gynecology
Attending, Obstetrics and Gynecology
Medical University of South Carolina
Charleston, South Carolina

**Series Editors:**

***Benjamin Clyburn, MD***
Assistant Professor of Medicine
Internal Medicine Residency Program Director
Medical University of South Carolina
Charleston, South Carolina

***George J. Taylor, MD***
Professor of Medicine
Medical University of South Carolina
Charleston, South Carolina

**Blackwell**
Publishing

Blackwell Publishing, Inc., 350 Main Street, Malden, Massachusetts 02148-5018, USA
Blackwell Science Ltd, Osney Mead, Oxford OX2 0EL, UK
Blackwell Science Asia Pty Ltd, 550 Swanston Street, Carlton South, Victoria 3053, Australia
Blackwell Verlag GmbH, Kurfürstendamm 57, 10707 Berlin, Germany



02 03 04 05 5 4 3 2 1

ISBN: 0-632-04664-3

Library of Congress Cataloging-in-Publication Data

Sleepwell. Volume 2, Surgery and obstetrics & gynecology/edited by E. Douglas Norcross, Paige R. Gernt.
p. ; cm.
ISBN 0-632-04664-3 (pbk.)
1. Obstetrics—Examinations, questions, etc. 2. Gynecology—Examinations, questions, etc. 3. Surgery—Examinations, questions, etc. 4. Physicians—Licenses—United States—Examinations—Study guides. I. Norcross, E. Douglas. II. Gernt, Paige R. III. Title: Surgery and obstetrics & gynecology. IV. Title: Surgery and obstetrics and gynecology.

[DNLM: 1. Surgical Procedures, Operative—Examination Questions. 2. Gynecology—Examination Questions. 3. Obstetrics—Examination Questions. WO 18.2 S6322 2002]
RG111.S58 2002
617'.0076–dc21

2002009535

A catalogue record for this title is available from the British Library

Acquisitions: Beverly Copland
Development: Angela Gagliano
Production: Debra Lally
Cover design: Leslie Haimes
Interior design: Mary McKeon
Typesetter: Techbooks in York, PA
Printed and bound by Sheridan Books in Ann Arbor, MI

For further information on Blackwell Publishing, visit our website:
www.medirect.com

**Notice:** The indications and dosages of all drugs in this book have been recommended in the medical literature and conform to the practices of the general community. The medications described and treatment prescriptions suggested do not necessarily have specific approval by the Food and Drug Administration for use in the diseases and dosages for which they are recommended. The package insert for each drug should be consulted for use and dosage as approved by the FDA. Because standards for usage change, it is advisable to keep abreast of revised recommendations, particularly those concerning new drugs.

# Contents

# Contributors


**William T. Adamson, MD**
Assistant Professor of Surgery and Pediatrics
Medical University of South Carolina
Attending Pediatric Surgeon
Medical University Hospital
Charleston, South Carolina

**Byron N. Bailey, MD**
Assistant Professor of Neurosurgery
Medical University of South Carolina
Attending Neurosurgeon
Medical University Hospital
Charleston, South Carolina

**Carlton C. Barnett, MD**
Assistant Professor of Surgery
Medical University of South Carolina
Attending Surgeon
Medical University Hospital
Charleston, South Carolina

**Thomas Brothers, MD, FACS**
Associate Professor of Surgery
Medical University of South Carolina
Attending Surgeon
Medical University Hospital
Charleston, South Carolina

**T. Karl Byrne, MD, FACS**
Associate Professor of Surgery
Medical University of South Carolina
Attending Surgeon
Medical University Hospital
Charleston, South Carolina

**Arthur J. Crumbley III, MD, FACS**
Associate Professor of Surgery
Medical University of South Carolina
Attending Cardiothoracic Surgeon
Medical University Hospital
Charleston, South Carolina

**Harry A. Demos, MD**
Assistant Professor of Orthopedic Surgery
Medical University of South Carolina
Attending Orthopedic Surgeon
Medical University Hospital
Charleston, South Carolina

**Paige R. Gernt, MD**
Assistant Professor of Obstetrics and Gynecology
Attending, Obstetrics and Gynecology
Medical University of South Carolina
Charleston, South Carolina

**William E. Gillanders, MD**
Assistant Professor of Surgery
Medical University of South Carolina
Attending Surgeon
Medical University Hospital
Charleston, South Carolina

**Charles N. Landen, Jr., MD**
Instructor in Obstetrics and Gynecology
Attending in Obstetrics and Gynecology
University of South Carolina School of Medicine
Columbia, South Carolina
Post-Doctoral Fellow, Microbiology and Immunology
Medical University of South Carolina
Charleston, South Carolina

**Angello Lin, MD**
Assistant Professor of Surgery
Medical University of South Carolina
Attending Surgeon
Medical University Hospital
Charleston, South Carolina

**Jobe C. Metts III, MD**
Assistant Professor of Urology
Medical University of South Carolina
Attending Urologist
Medical University Hospital
Charleston, South Carolina

**E. Douglas Norcross, MD, FACS**
Associate Professor of Surgery
Medical University of South Carolina
Attending Surgeon
Medical University Hospital
Charleston, South Carolina

**Patrick J. O'Neill, MD**
Assistant Professor of Surgery
Medical University of South Carolina
Attending Plastic Surgeon
Medical University Hospital
Charleston, South Carolina

**Jay G. Robison, MD, FACS**
Associate Professor of Vascular Surgery
Medical University of South Carolina
Attending Surgeon
Medical University Hospital
Charleston, South Carolina

**Mitchell J. Siegan, MD**
Assistant Professor of Anesthesiology
Medical University of South Carolina
Charleston, South Carolina
Attending Anesthesiologist
Grand Strand Regional Medical Center
Myrtle Beach, South Carolina

# Reviewers

**Carol Cox, MD**
Chief Resident in Obstetrics & Gynecology
University of South Florida
Tampa, Florida

**Ernest Han, MD**
Resident in Obstetrics & Gynecology
Women and Infants Hospital
Providence, Rhode Island

**Pedram Ilbeigi, DO**
Resident in Surgery
University of Medicine & Dentistry of New Jersey
Newark, New Jersey

**Matthew F. Kalady, MD**
Resident in General Surgery
Duke University Medical Center
Durham, North Carolina

**Robert Kim, MD**
Resident in Obstetrics & Gynecology
Northwestern University
Chicago, Illinois

**Solange Pendas, MD**
Surgical Oncology Fellow
City of Hope National Medical Center
Duarte, California

**Timothy Tsui, MD**
Chief Resident
Cedars-Sinai Medical Center
Los Angeles, California

**Donald Yarbrough, MD**
Resident in Surgery
Mayo Clinic
Cleveland, Ohio

# • Preface

The *SleepWell Review* series is a **review for the National Board examinations,** compiled for students and residents taking parts 2 and 3 as well as international medical graduates. It is also **suitable for recertification exams in family medicine and state licensure exams.**

In the three volumes, we have attempted to cover all of the topics that you will encounter on the exams. The series differs from many practice tests, as we provide a brief discussion of the questions and answers. The emphasis is on "brief," and we do not pretend that the discussions provide a thorough review—you do not have time for that. Rather, the short explanations will remind you of the concept(s) that the board examiner wants you to know. Understand that clinical issue and you will be able to handle related questions.

Many of you will use this review as a study guide as you begin preparing for the boards. For the brave soul who decides not to study, it would be a suitable one-shot review. For most of you, we suggest using it just before the exam. After studying for months, you are burned out and cannot memorize another table or list of facts. So what do you do in the last week? Here is our best advice: go to the gym every day, get to bed early and breeze through these sample questions with their short explanations. **Use these books** as your last study exercise, and **you will sleep well the night before the boards.**

We welcome feedback and suggestions you may have on this book or any in the new *SleepWell Review* series. Send to blue@blacksci.com.

# • Section 1

# Surgery

William T. Adamson, MD
Byron N. Bailey, MD
Carlton C. Barnett, MD
Thomas Brothers, MD, FACS
T. Karl Byrne, MD, FACS
Arthur J. Crumbley III, MD, FACS
Harry A. Demos, MD
William E. Gillanders, MD
Angello Lin, MD
Jobe C. Metts III, MD
E. Douglas Norcross, MD, FACS
Patrick J. O'Neill, MD
Jay G. Robinson, MD, FACS
Mitchell J. Siegan, MD

## CASE PRESENTATION

You are on call for the emergency department when a 22-year-old man is brought to the hospital after sustaining a single gunshot wound to the left thigh. On examination, there is an entrance wound on the anterior thigh medial to the femur. No exit wound is identified. Upon removing the dressing placed by pre-hospital personnel, pulsatile bleeding comes from the wound. This is being controlled with direct manual pressure. The patient is awake and alert and is complaining of pain in his injured leg. Blood pressure is 70/30, and his pulse rate is 135.

1. Initial stabilization should include:
   A. Endotracheal intubation
   B. Insertion of triple-lumen central venous catheter
   C. Placement of two 16-gauge peripheral IVs
   D. Placement of clamps in wound to control hemorrhage
   E. Placement of a tourniquet on the injured thigh
2. The IV fluid of choice in this patient is:
   A. Quarter-normal saline solution
   B. Lactated Ringer's solution
   C. Hespan
   D. Half-normal (0.45) saline solution with 20 mEq KCl per liter
   E. 5% albumin solution
3. After initial stabilization, the next step in the patient's management would be to:
   A. Arrange for an arteriogram of the injured leg in the angiography suite
   B. Take the patient immediately to the operating room for surgical exploration
   C. Perform a bedside single-film arteriogram in the emergency department
   D. Perform a Doppler study of the arteries of the injured leg
   E. Probe the wound to determine the path of the bullet
4. Following initial evaluation and stabilization, the patient is taken to surgery. An injury to the superficial femoral artery is identified and repaired with a reversed saphenous vein graft. Four hours postoperatively, the patient is complaining of severe pain in his lower leg. On examination, pulses are present but somewhat diminished. Passive stretch of the great toe results in severe pain in the back of the patient's calf. The leg is edematous. The next step in management is:
   A. Immediate arteriogram in the angiography suite
   B. Doppler study of arterial supply to the injured leg
   C. Bedside single-film arteriogram
   D. Measurement of blood pressure in the affected leg
   E. Measurement of pressures in the leg's fascial compartments

## COMMENT

**Initial resuscitation of hemorrhagic shock** • In this case, the patient presented in hemorrhagic shock. With no airway compromise, intubation is not necessary. Manual pressure on the wound will control bleeding. Placement of clamps in the wound without proper exposure may result in damage to other structures and is to be avoided. Tourniquets are rarely necessary and put the limb at risk. Resuscitation is best accomplished with large-bore peripheral intravenous access rather than with long, smaller-bore central venous lines.

**Resuscitation fluids** • The fluid of choice for resuscitation of hemorrhagic shock is an isotonic crystalloid solution (normal saline or lactated Ringer's solution). Colloid solutions have no demonstrable advantage over crystalloid solutions but are substantially more expensive and, in the case of albumin solutions, carry some risk of disease transmission.

**Decision making in penetrating extremity trauma** • The management of penetrating injuries in the vicinity of major vessels has changed significantly over the past several years. In the past, patients with "hard signs" of vascular injury underwent mandatory exploration, while those with "soft signs," including injury path in proximity to a major vessel, underwent arteriography. It is now apparent that in the presence of hard signs (active bleeding, large or expanding hematoma, thrill or bruit, or signs of distal ischemia), patients should go immediately to the operating room without further workup. Exceptions include shotgun injuries in which the exact location of injury cannot be determined. Angiography would be indicated in this group of patients.

If no hard signs are present, it is generally felt that no further workup is required. In many institutions, such patients are discharged from the emergency department with instructions to return if any signs of ischemia develop and with appropriate follow-up. Development of late ischemia in these patients is rare.

**Compartment syndrome** • This patient has developed a compartment syndrome. Muscle swelling—which can occur within a day of injury—causes increased pressure within the fascial compartment, which compromises arterial flow. Loss of pulses is a late sign, as are neurologic deficits. Early recognition is critical for limb salvage. Measurement of compartment pressures will make the diagnosis and should be performed early. Once identified, immediate fasciotomy is essential.

**Answers** • 1-C 2-B 3-B 4-E

## CASE PRESENTATION

A patient is brought to the emergency department of a small community hospital after a severe motor vehicle collision. He is unconscious but has purposeful (withdrawal) response to painful stimuli, and the right pupil is larger than the left. His initial blood pressure is 80/30 and his pulse is 120 beats per minute. He has obvious deformities of the left femur and left forearm suggestive of fractures. Chest radiograph reveals multiple rib fractures on the left. A pelvis x-ray is unremarkable. The patient's abdomen is distended and intra-abdominal bleeding is suspected. His blood pressure rises to 130/85 after 2 liters of Ringer's lactate solution is administered, but he requires ongoing fluid resuscitation to maintain this blood pressure. Although there are general surgeons on call, there is no neurosurgeon on the hospital staff.

1. Best management includes:
   - A. Stabilization and transfer to the nearest hospital with a neurosurgeon capable of providing the care needed by the patient
   - B. Exploratory laparotomy to control bleeding if blood pressure is unstable and intra-abdominal bleeding is identified.
   - C. X-rays of the left femur and left forearm and CT scan of the head before transfer
   - D. A and B
2. Which of the following is true about evaluation of this patient's abdomen?
   - A. Abdominal evaluation is not indicated in this patient.
   - B. CT scan would have a higher sensitivity in the detection of intra-abdominal hemorrhage than diagnostic peritoneal lavage.
   - C. Ultrasound would be sufficient to diagnose the source of any intra-abdominal hemorrhage identified.
   - D. CT scan may identify injuries that could be treated nonoperatively.
   - E. Diagnostic peritoneal lavage will identify retroperitoneal injury.
3. The most likely cause of hypotension in this patient is:
   - A. Spinal cord injury
   - B. Brain injury
   - C. Blood loss
   - D. Infection
   - E. Cardiac injury

## COMMENT

**Interhospital transfer of the injured patient** • The seriously injured patient is best treated at a facility capable of providing a full spectrum of injury care with full subspecialty support. Patients should be transferred to such a facility as soon as they are stable enough for transfer, or at least stabilized to the greatest extent possible at the referring hospital. Prior to transfer, the patient's airway must be secured, oxygenation and ventilation stabilized, clinically apparent fractures splinted, and the patient's spine protected on a long spine board with a semirigid cervical collar. Finally, the patient must be stabilized hemodynamically. This cannot be accomplished in the face of ongoing hemorrhage. In this case, the patient requires ongoing fluid resuscitation, suggesting ongoing intra-abdominal bleeding. Exploratory laparotomy should be performed to stop this bleeding prior to transfer. No testing should be performed that is not going to be acted on at the referring hospital. Therefore, CT scans of the brain, radiographs of the extremities, and so forth are not necessary prior to transfer and only delay transfer.

**Evaluation of the abdomen in blunt trauma** • Physical examination alone is unreliable in many patients with traumatic injuries. Therefore, other methods must often be employed. Indications include closed head injury, need for prolonged anesthesia, abdominal pain or tenderness, hypotension, spinal cord injury, and alcohol- or drug-related intoxication. Diagnostic peritoneal lavage has a very high sensitivity but has the disadvantages of being invasive, of not evaluating the retroperitoneum, and of being unable to identify the actual site or severity of organ injury. Ultrasound shares these disadvantages. It is, however, noninvasive. CT scan allows for identification of the actual site of injury and assessment of its severity, allowing the clinician to evaluate the feasibility of employing nonoperative management strategies.

**Causes of shock in the injured patient** • Hypotension in a recently injured patient is most commonly the result of hemorrhage. Head injury, up to the point of herniation, usually causes hypertension and bradycardia. Spinal cord injury may lead to loss of sympathetic innervation below the level of the injury. The resulting hypotension is associated with bradycardia. Cardiac injury resulting in hypotension is rare. Sepsis would not likely be a factor acutely.

**Answers** • 1-D 2-D 3-C

## CASE PRESENTATION

A 35-year-old man is brought to the hospital after falling from a ladder. He is reported to have landed on his head. He is initially unconscious but is combative when medics arrive at the scene. He remains hemodynamically stable throughout transport.

1. Which of the following statements about epidural hematoma is true?
   A. Epidural hematoma is more commonly associated with underlying brain injury than subdural hematoma.
   B. Epidural hematoma characteristically is convex on the side of the skull and concave on the side of the brain.
   C. Even with rapid treatment, epidural hematoma carries a worse neurologic prognosis than subdural hematoma.
   D. A lucid interval is characteristic of epidural hematoma.
   E. Epidural hematomas are always associated with injury to the middle meningeal artery.
2. Evaluation reveals a cerebral contusion with surrounding edema and a slight midline shift. Which of the following parameters would require alterations in the treatment of this patient?
   A. Pulmonary artery wedge pressure of 9 mm Hg
   B. Intracranial pressure (ICP) of 26 mm Hg with a mean arterial pressure (MAP) of 80 mm Hg
   C. $Pao_2$ equal to 98 mm Hg
   D. $Paco_2$ equal to 36 mm Hg
   E. Hemoglobin concentration of 11 g/dL
3. Which of the following would be consistent with cerebral death (brain death)?
   A. Loss of the "doll's eyes" response
   B. Loss of the corneal reflex
   C. Presence of the patellar reflex
   D. Apnea in the presence of an elevated $Paco_2$
   E. All of the above

## COMMENT

**Epidural hematoma** • Epidural hematoma most commonly results from injuries to the vessels of the meninges and skull. While damage to the middle meningeal artery is a common source of these hematomas, it is not the only source. Because these lesions are largely the result of injuries to the meninges and skull rather than injuries to the brain itself, they have a better prognosis when rapidly and appropriately treated. Characteristically, these lesions are biconvex in shape. A lucid interval is often described as, after the brief initial loss of consciousness, the clot enlarges and pressure within the cranial vault increases, resulting in a secondary loss of consciousness.

**Management of closed head injury** • The treatment of closed head injury centers around assuring survival of areas of injured brain and avoiding further brain cell death in these damaged regions. To accomplish this, oxygen and nutrient delivery to, and removal of waste products from, the injured brain must be optimized. Maintenance of oxygen delivery depends on adequate hemoglobin levels, adequate hemoglobin saturation, and adequate cardiac output.

Maintenance of normal intravascular volume (as measured by pulmonary artery wedge pressure) is desirable. Dehydration may result in decreased cardiac filling and decreased cardiac output and, therefore, decreased perfusion of the injured brain. Volume overload, on the other hand, can result in cerebral swelling and increases in intracranial pressure with a resultant decrease in perfusion. Hyperventilation, which may potentially lower intracranial pressure, does so at the expense of reduced blood flow to the injured brain. Although commonly employed in the past, it is now clear that vigorous hyperventilation should be avoided.

Outcomes of closed head injury are better when cerebral perfusion pressure (mean arterial pressure minus intracranial pressure) is higher than 70 mm Hg. Low cerebral perfusion pressure demands immediate measures to lower ICP or increase MAP.

**Brain death** • An evaluation of brain death requires that all functions of the brain and brainstem have ceased. Loss of doll's eyes response, failure to respond to cold caloric testing, fixed dilated pupils, and apnea all occur in this condition. Pure spinal reflexes (i.e., the deep tendon reflexes) may remain intact because they do not require input from the brain.

**Answers** • 1-D 2-B 3-E

## CASE PRESENTATION

A 68-year-old patient in the intensive care unit develops hypotension.

1. Which of the following would be most consistent with hypovolemic shock?
   A. Elevated cardiac index measurement with low systemic vascular resistance
   B. Decreased cardiac index with increased systemic vascular resistance
   C. Bradycardia and decreased right atrial pressure
   D. Bradycardia and increased right atrial pressure
   E. Tachycardia and increased pulmonary artery wedge pressure
2. Which of the following would be most consistent with cardiogenic shock due to acute myocardial infarction?
   A. Elevated cardiac index measurement with low systemic vascular resistance
   B. Decreased cardiac index with decreased systemic vascular resistance
   C. Bradycardia and decreased right atrial pressure
   D. Bradycardia and increased right atrial pressure
   E. Tachycardia and increased pulmonary artery wedge pressure
3. Which of the following would be most consistent with neurogenic (spinal) shock?
   A. Elevated cardiac index measurement with low systemic vascular resistance
   B. Decreased cardiac index with increased systemic vascular resistance
   C. Bradycardia and decreased right atrial pressure
   D. Bradycardia and increased right atrial pressure
   E. Tachycardia and increased pulmonary artery wedge pressure
4. Which of the following would be most consistent with septic shock?
   A. Elevated cardiac index measurement with low systemic vascular resistance
   B. Decreased cardiac index with increased systemic vascular resistance
   C. Bradycardia and decreased right atrial pressure
   D. Bradycardia and increased right atrial pressure
   E. Tachycardia and increased pulmonary artery wedge pressure

## COMMENT

**Hypovolemic shock** • Hemodynamic differences in the various shock states can be used to help determine the etiology of the hypotension. Hemorrhagic and hypovolemic shock result from the loss of blood or fluid from the intravascular space. Compensatory mechanisms include increased output from the sympathetic nervous system. This results in an increase in vascular tone and vascular resistance, and tachycardia. With hypovolemia, cardiac filling pressures (both right atrial and pulmonary wedge pressure) are low.

**Cardiogenic shock** • Like hemorrhagic shock, cardiogenic shock is associated with output from the sympathetic nervous system. However, vascular volume is normal. Pump failure results in increases in cardiac filling pressures as ejection fraction decreases (fraction decreases and the kidneys retain sodium and water in response to diminished renal perfusion).

**Spinal shock** • Spinal shock is caused by a loss of sympathetic tone. The normal tonic parasympathetic output to the heart remains unopposed, with a resultant bradycardia. Loss of vascular tone in the arterial circulation results in a decrease in systemic vascular resistance, while pooling of blood in the capacitance vessels diminishes cardiac filling with a fall in right-sided cardiac filling pressures.

**Septic shock** • Septic shock is a complex manifestation of a diffuse systemic inflammatory response with a number of possible inciting causes. In its initial stages, it is associated with a loss of vascular tone and decreased systemic vascular resistance, with a simultaneous increase in cardiac output. These patients are often febrile and display other manifestations of organ insufficiency or organ failure.

**Answers** • 1-B 2-E 3-C 4-A

## CASE PRESENTATION

A 74-year-old man had an elective right hemicolectomy to remove a large villous adenoma. The procedure was difficult because of the presence of dense adhesions in the abdomen from a previous abdominal aortic aneurysm repair. In the recovery room, the patient develops hypotension and tachycardia. Urine output decreases significantly. His hemoglobin concentration at the start of the case was 13 g/dL. A repeat measurement in the recovery room drawn at the time the patient first became hypotensive reveals a hemoglobin concentration of 11.5 g/dL. Intraoperative blood loss during the procedure was estimated to be 500 mL. ECG is unremarkable, and heart sounds are normal except for a preexisting grade 2 diastolic murmur. Chest x-ray is clear.

1. The most likely cause of the patient's hypotension and tachycardia is:
   A. Myocardial infarction
   B. Pulmonary embolus
   C. Tension pneumothorax
   D. Intra-abdominal hemorrhage
   E. Air embolus
2. After appropriate stabilization, the patient is taken to the intensive care unit. On postoperative day 6, large amounts of a brownish fluid are seen coming from the wound. He is afebrile. This is characteristic of which of the following?
   A. Fascial dehiscence
   B. *Staphylococcus aureus* wound infection
   C. Small-bowel fistula
   D. Leak of ascitic fluid
   E. *Pseudomonas aeruginosa* wound infection
3. Over the next several days the patient's respiratory status deteriorates. Which of the following is most consistent with adult respiratory distress syndrome (ARDS) as a cause for this deterioration?
   A. Normal chest x-ray, increased pulmonary artery pressure, and tachypnea
   B. Chest x-ray with a unilateral infiltrate, increased alveolar-arterial oxygen gradient (A-a gradient), and tachypnea
   C. Diffuse infiltrates on chest x-ray, abnormally elevated pulmonary artery wedge pressure (24 mm Hg), and tachypnea
   D. Diffuse infiltrates on chest x-ray, normal pulmonary artery wedge pressure (12 mm Hg), and tachypnea
   E. Normal chest x-ray, increased $Paco_2$, and normal A-a gradient

## COMMENT

**Postoperative hypovolemia** • Early postoperative hypotension should always alert one to the possibility of bleeding. Although the other etiologies listed can be considered, bleeding is most common. The hemoglobin concentration can be deceiving, because it will not fall with acute blood loss. As intravascular volume is replaced with saline (fluid resuscitation), there will be hemodilution with a fall in the hemoglobin concentration as lost blood is replaced by other fluids. Rapid and unresuscitated blood loss will not initially cause a fall in hemoglobin concentration.

**Fascial dehiscence** • Brown fluid coming from an abdominal wound in the early postoperative period should make a clinician suspicious of a disruption of the fascial closure. Wound infections generally occur about 1 week postoperatively and may ultimately lead to fascial dehiscence. However, these are usually associated with fever and redness of the skin around the wound. Pus is generally present. This patient has no clear etiology for ascites that was not present preoperatively. Ascitic fluid is usually serous rather than brown.

**Adult respiratory distress syndrome** • ARDS is the result of injury to the alveolar-capillary membrane, allowing exudation of fluid and protein into alveoli. This pulmonary manifestation of systemic inflammation is not localized to any one area of the lung. Noncardiac pulmonary edema can be distinguished from the edema of left ventricular failure by measuring the pulmonary wedge pressure (the LV filling pressure). When elevated, the diagnosis is heart failure. When less than 20 mm Hg, the diffuse infiltrates are from ARDS. Patients with ARDS will develop tachypnea and have an increased gradient between the partial pressure of oxygen in their alveoli and the partial pressure of oxygen in their arterial blood (increased A-a gradient).

**Answers** • 1-D 2-A 3-D

## CASE PRESENTATION

A 25-year-old woman presents to the emergency department with sudden onset of moderately severe abdominal pain.

1. The patient describes the pain as severe and unrelenting. It does not seem to wax or wane in intensity. Constant pain suggests which of the following disorders?
   A. Acute appendicitis
   B. Superior mesenteric artery occlusion
   C. Perforated ulcer
   D. Ruptured sigmoid colon diverticulum
   E. Any of the above
2. The pain originated at the umbilicus but, over the past several hours, has moved to the right lower quadrant. Which of the following is consistent with the diagnosis of acute appendicitis?
   A. Low-grade fever
   B. Loss of appetite
   C. Pain in the right lower quadrant of the abdomen with palpation in the left lower quadrant of the abdomen
   D. Diarrhea
   E. A, B, and C
3. A decision is made to perform surgery through a right lower quadrant abdominal incision. At the time of surgery, the appendix is noted to be normal. However, the distal ileum is inflamed. There is no evidence of obstruction or perforation. The cecum is not involved in this process. Appropriate management would be:
   A. End the procedure and close all incisions
   B. Perform an appendectomy
   C. Perform a small-bowel resection to include the inflamed bowel
   D. Create a loop ileostomy proximal to the area of inflammation
   E. Perform a small-bowel resection and remove the appendix
4. Which of the following may result from resection of the terminal ileum?
   A. Vitamin $B_{12}$ deficiency
   B. Iron deficiency
   C. Calcium deficiency
   D. All of the above
   E. None of the above

## COMMENT

**Abdominal pain fibers** • Visceral pain receptors respond to ischemia and stretch, whereas pain receptors within the parietal peritoneum respond to inflammation. Colicky pain is caused by increasing distension of hollow viscera resulting from proximal peristalsis, usually against a point of obstruction. Thus, this patient's constant pain is not consistent with early small-bowel obstruction. Ischemic pain and the pain from parietal peritoneal irritation are constant, so it is not waves of peristalsis causing the pain. Superior mesenteric artery occlusion, perforated duodenal ulcer, acute appendicitis, and peritonitis from a perforated diverticulum all would produce constant pain.

**Acute appendicitis** • Classically, uncomplicated acute appendicitis is accompanied by decreased appetite, low-grade fever, a moderately increased white blood cell count, and occasionally one or two episodes of vomiting. Diarrhea is unusual and suggests infection or inflammation of the bowel rather than appendicitis.

Initially, the pain of acute appendicitis is caused by obstruction of the appendiceal lumen, which becomes distended. The visceral pain fibers, which localize pain from the midgut structures, including the appendix, to the area of the umbilicus, are stimulated by this distension. However, peristalsis is minimal, so cramping pain is not typical. As the surface of the appendix becomes inflamed, surrounding parietal peritoneal nerves are stimulated. These nerves are able to accurately localize pain. The pain, therefore, moves to the area overlying the appendix in the right lower quadrant of the abdomen. *Rovsing's sign* is the production of pain in the right lower quadrant with pressure in the left lower quadrant. It is caused by movement of the parietal peritoneum in the right lower quadrant as pressure is applied in the left lower quadrant.

**The normal appendix during surgery for right lower quadrant abdominal pain** • In the event that appendicitis is not identified at the time of surgery, it is important to search for other causes, in this case terminal ileitis. Since no treatment has been initiated for this condition, and since the condition may respond to medical therapy without the need for ileal resection, the small bowel generally is not removed unless some associated complication such as fistula, perforation, or obstruction is identified. Because ileitis may be a recurrent problem, many would remove the appendix to avoid future confusion (experienced surgeons argue this both ways).

**Side effects of ileal resection** • Resection of the terminal ileum can have a number of effects. Vitamin $B_{12}$ is absorbed in the terminal ileum, as are bile salts. Loss of this segment of the bowel may result in vitamin $B_{12}$ deficiency. Bile salts passing into the colon can cause diarrhea. The loss of the normal enterohepatic circulation can result in bile salt depletion and fat malabsorption. Iron absorption and calcium absorption tend to occur largely in the proximal small bowel.

**Answers** • 1-E 2-E 3-A or B 4-A

## CASE PRESENTATION

A 37-year-old, 50-kg woman is brought to the emergency department 2 hours after being pulled from a burning house trailer. She is unresponsive, tachycardic, and mildly hypotensive. She has full-thickness (third-degree) burns to her posterior torso as well as circumferentially around her entire right arm. Her left arm has partial-thickness (second-degree) burns throughout.

1. Approximately what percentage of her body surface area is burned?
   A. 9%
   B. 18%
   C. 27%
   D. 36%
   E. 45%
2. Lactated Ringer's solution is initiated. What would be the most appropriate rate at which to begin fluid resuscitation in this patient?
   A. 125 cc/hr
   B. 300 cc/hr
   C. 450 cc/hr
   D. 600 cc/hr
   E. 750 cc/hr
3. Which of the following would be expected if carbon monoxide poisoning was the cause of her altered mental status?
   A. $Pa_{O_2}$ equals 90 mm Hg on room air (normal 80–100 mm Hg)
   B. Hemoglobin saturation of 100% measured by pulse oximetry
   C. Metabolic acidosis
   D. All of the above
   E. None of the above
4. Silver sulfadiazine (Silvadene) cream is applied to the burn wounds. To monitor for complications of this agent, which of the following laboratory tests must be ordered?
   A. Serum potassium level
   B. Serum bicarbonate level
   C. Hemoglobin concentration
   D. Serum creatinine level
   E. White blood cell count

## COMMENT

**Estimating burn size** • Burn wound resuscitation begins with estimation of the size of the burn wound. The rule of nines is a commonly employed method to evaluate the percentage of the body surface area burned. The head and each arm are each estimated to account for 9% of the body surface area. The front of the torso, the back of the torso, and the left leg and right leg are each considered to contain 18% of the total body surface area. The genitalia make up the last 1% of the body surface area.

**Fluid resuscitation of the burn patient** • Initial fluid requirements are most commonly estimated using the *Parkland formula*. According to this formula, the total requirement of lactated Ringer's solution in the first 24 hours after injury is 4 cc/kg per percent body surface area burned (for second- and third-degree burns). Half of that volume is administered in the first 8 hours after injury. In this case, it is administered over a 6-hour period because 2 hours had already passed before the patient arrived in the emergency department following injury.

**Carbon monoxide poisoning** • Carbon monoxide poisoning should always be considered in patients trapped in an enclosed space during a fire. Carbon monoxide binds to the hemoglobin molecule in place of oxygen. The resultant decrease in oxygen delivery to the tissues may result in metabolic acidosis due to the development of anaerobic metabolism and lactate production. Pulse oximeters measure the color of the blood to calculate hemoglobin saturation. Because the hemoglobin's oxygen binding sites are filled, the hemoglobin assumes the "red" color of fully oxygenated hemoglobin, causing misleading pulse oximeter readings. Dissolved oxygen content is not affected, making arterial blood gas analysis, which measures the partial pressure exerted by dissolved gases in the blood, unable to detect the abnormality. Whenever carbon monoxide poisoning is suspected, a carboxyhemoglobin level should be obtained.

**Side effects of topical antibiotics used in burn care** • Topical antimicrobials remain an important part of burn wound management to prevent deep burn wound infection. They are not without potential complications, however. Silver sulfadiazine cream can cause neutropenia. Mafenide acetate is a carbonic anhydrase inhibitor. Its use can cause a metabolic acidosis.

**Answers** • 1-D 2-D 3-D 4-E

## CASE PRESENTATION

A 63-year-old man with no chronic medical problems presents to the emergency department with a 2-day history of intermittent abdominal pain and vomiting. He reports that he has not had a bowel movement since the pain started and he has passed no flatus in the past 24 hours. Abdominal x-rays reveal distended loops of small intestine with no air in the colon.

1. The most likely additional history is:
   A. A mass in the scrotum
   B. Previous abdominal surgery
   C. Weight loss over the past 3 months
   D. Diarrhea
   E. Jaundice
2. Physical examination reveals hyperactive bowel sounds with occasional "rushes" associated with episodes of pain as well as abdominal tenderness. Laboratory evaluation reveals an elevated white blood cell count and a slightly elevated serum amylase level. The best course of management at this time would be which of the following?
   A. Place a nasogastric tube and admit for repeated abdominal evaluations.
   B. Schedule the patient for an upper gastrointestinal contrast study with small-bowel follow-through.
   C. Schedule an abdominal CT scan.
   D. Schedule a superior mesenteric artery arteriogram.
   E. Schedule the patient for exploratory laparotomy.
3. The patient is, at the appropriate time, taken to surgery. At exploration a mass is identified in the mid jejunum. The most likely benign neoplasm is:
   A. Leiomyoma
   B. Hemangioma
   C. Fibroma
   D. Lipoma
   E. Adenomatous polyp
4. The tumor is resected and found to be malignant. The most likely diagnosis is:
   A. Lymphoma
   B. Carcinoid tumor
   C. Adenocarcinoma
   D. Leiomyosarcoma
   E. Lymphangioma

## COMMENT

**Causes of small-bowel obstruction** • The patient has symptoms characteristic of complete small-bowel obstruction. Historical details that would suggest partial obstruction include continued passage of flatus or stool more than approximately 6 hours after onset of symptoms. Abdominal x-rays revealing air in the distal colon more than about 6 to 12 hours after the onset of symptoms are also suggestive of partial small-bowel obstruction. The most common cause of this condition is adhesions from previous abdominal surgery. Hernias, inflammatory bowel disease, and metastatic or primary neoplasms are less common.

**Indications for surgery in small-bowel obstruction** • In this case, there are clear suggestions of complete obstruction. This places the patient at risk for strangulation and bowel ischemia. Signs of strangulated obstruction include continuous rather than intermittent pain; fever; tachycardia; evidence of peritoneal irritation; leukocytosis; and moderate elevations of serum amylase level. However, these signs have low sensitivity and low specificity for strangulation. Therefore, any patient with acceptable operative risk displaying signs of complete small-bowel obstruction is best treated with urgent exploration. Further diagnostic testing adds little to the decision-making process, and observation in this setting carries a risk of bowel strangulation, ischemia, or perforation.

**Benign small-bowel tumors** • Lymphangioma is an uncommon benign small-bowel tumor. Among the other benign small-bowel tumors, leiomyomas are most common (30% to 40% of small-bowel benign tumors). Adenomatous polyps (20% to 30%), lipomas (15% to 20% of small-bowel benign tumors), hemangiomas (<10%), and fibromas (<5%), are also benign neoplasms found in the small bowel.

**Malignant small-bowel tumors** • Primary small-bowel tumors are far less common than tumors of the large bowel. The most common malignant tumors are adenocarcinoma (40% to 50% of small-bowel malignancies), carcinoid tumor (20% to 30% of small-bowel malignancies), lymphoma (20% to 25% of small-bowel malignancies), and leiomyosarcoma, which is also known as a gastrointestinal stromal tumor (10% to 15% of small-bowel malignancies).

**Answers** • 1-B 2-E 3-A 4-C

## CASE PRESENTATION

You are called to see a 78-year-old woman with abdominal pain that begins 1 hour after meals. Her symptoms have been present for the past 6 months. The pain is located in the mid abdomen and feels like a dull ache. It gradually subsides and then recurs with subsequent meals. The patient has had a 30-pound weight loss over the past several months. Her past medical history is significant for a myocardial infarction with a subsequent coronary artery bypass operation. She has also undergone a femoral popliteal arterial bypass.

1. Which of the following tests is most likely to reveal the diagnosis?
   A. Ultrasound examination of the gall bladder
   B. Serum amylase measurement
   C. Arteriogram
   D. Upper gastrointestinal contrast study with small-bowel follow-through
   E. Abdominal CT scan
2. Two weeks later the patient presents to the emergency room with severe abdominal pain. She describes the pain as unremitting and severe. On physical examination, she has little abdominal wall tenderness or guarding. Palpation does not identify any mass or areas of unusual tenderness. Her lungs are clear and her heart has no audible murmur. Her pulse is irregular and she is hypotensive. Laboratory examination reveals a profound metabolic acidosis. Abdominal plain x-rays are unremarkable. The next step in her management would be:
   A. Abdominal CT scan
   B. Arteriogram
   C. Upper gastrointestinal contrast study with small-bowel follow-through
   D. Exploratory laparotomy
   E. Endoscopic retrograde cholangiopancreatography
3. A decision is made to take the patient to surgery. A massive small-bowel resection is performed, leaving her with only 30 cm of small bowel. She is placed on total parenteral nutrition and is discharged from the hospital. Which of the following would be a recognized complication for a patient with this condition?
   A. Cholelithiasis
   B. Hepatic failure
   C. Peptic ulcer disease
   D. Ureteral calculi
   E. All of the above

## COMMENT

**Evaluation of intestinal angina** • This patient demonstrates symptoms consistent with chronic mesenteric ischemia. This is almost always the result of atherosclerotic occlusive disease. Passage of foodstuffs through the small bowel increases the work of the bowel. Because of the inability to increase flow in the diseased vessels, ischemia develops, causing pain after meals. Patients develop "food fear," resulting in weight loss. Mesenteric arteriography would reveal the vascular disease and is indicated in this patient.

**Management of mesenteric occlusion** • When the patient returns to the emergency department, she displays signs of acute mesenteric occlusion, possibly the result of an embolus from her heart (the irregular rhythm suggests atrial fibrillation) or superior mesenteric artery thrombosis. Early in the course of acute occlusion, arteriography may be useful. Infusion of thrombolytic agents, balloon dilatation, and placement of intravascular stents may alleviate the acute condition. However, this patient shows evidence of intestinal necrosis and hemodynamic decompensation. Operative intervention is mandatory.

**Short-bowel syndrome** • Massive small-bowel resection may result in short-bowel syndrome and malabsorption. Alterations in bile salt reabsorption change the composition of bile and can lead to gallstone formation. Long-term parenteral nutritional support can result in hepatic steatosis and ultimately hepatic insufficiency. Gastric acid hypersecretion is common, although usually transient. Nephrolithiasis is very common. Fat malabsorption may cause calcium to be bound to intraluminal fat. Oxalate is normally bound to calcium, preventing its absorption. Decreases in unbound intraluminal calcium result in increased oxalate absorption and formation of oxalate stones.

**Answers** • 1-C 2-D 3-E

## CASE PRESENTATION

A 31-year-old man complains of chronic diarrhea.

1. Which of the following comparisons between Crohn's disease and ulcerative colitis is true?
   A. Pain is more common in patients with ulcerative colitis.
   B. Gastrointestinal hemorrhage is more common in patients with Crohn's disease than in those with ulcerative colitis.
   C. Patients with ulcerative colitis, but not those with Crohn's disease, are at increased risk of malignancy compared with the general population.
   D. Crohn's disease is more commonly associated with discontinuous areas of inflammation than is ulcerative colitis, which is usually continuous.
   E. Crohn's disease is usually limited to the mucosal layer of the bowel, whereas ulcerative colitis more often involves the full thickness of the bowel wall.
2. Common indications for surgery in ulcerative colitis include:
   A. Diarrhea unresponsive to medical therapy
   B. Toxic megacolon
   C. Colonic mucosal dysplasia
   D. Fistula
   E. A, B, and C
3. Common indications for surgery in Crohn's disease include which of the following?
   A. Symptoms unresponsive to medical therapy
   B. Fistula
   C. Stricture
   D. Small-bowel obstruction
   E. All of the above
4. The patient undergoes a small-bowel resection. Prior to discharge, bilious fluid is noted to be coming from the wound. A small-bowel fistula is diagnosed on fluoroscopic evaluation. Which of the following is true?
   A. Enterocutaneous fistulas resulting from inflammatory bowel disease are more likely to close spontaneously than iatrogenic fistulas.
   B. Obstruction distal to the fistula delays, but does not usually prevent, spontaneous closure.
   C. Most fistulas that close spontaneously do so within the first 2 months.
   D. Inflammatory bowel disease is the most common cause of enterocutaneous fistula.
   E. Somatostatin administration has a significant effect on the rate of spontaneous fistula closure.

## COMMENT

**Characteristics of inflammatory bowel disease** • Inflammatory bowel disease is a spectrum of diseases that often resist exact characterization. Nonetheless, certain characteristics may help distinguish the two major components of this disease complex, Crohn's disease and ulcerative colitis. Crohn's disease is a full-thickness granulomatous inflammatory process that may involve the small bowel or the large bowel, often simultaneously and often in discontinuity. Diarrhea and abdominal pain are common symptoms of this disease process and, if unremitting despite aggressive medical therapy, may warrant resection of obviously involved bowel. Other complications that might mandate operative intervention include fistulas both to the skin and to other abdominal hollow viscera, acute intestinal obstruction, and chronic stricture formation. Bowel malignancy is more common in these patients than in the unaffected population but not to the same degree as in ulcerative colitis. Severe bleeding is an unusual complication in this disease.

**Indications for surgery in ulcerative colitis** • Ulcerative colitis is limited to the mucosal layer of the large intestine. The disease generally starts distally and progresses proximally without skipping segments, as may occur in Crohn's disease. Complications that may require colectomy include toxic megacolon and colonic malignancy. Because of this latter complication, careful screening for dysplasia with colonoscopic evaluation is very important. Many authors recommend prophylactic colectomy to avoid the very high risk of colon carcinoma. Certainly, any evidence of dysplasia warrants operative intervention. Massive hemorrhage is also a recognized complication and often occurs in conjunction with episodes of toxic megacolon. Life-threatening hemorrhage, although unusual, may be an indication for emergent colectomy. Diarrhea is an important symptom in these patients and, if unrelenting despite treatment, may require surgery. Pain is unusual in this condition. Since the full thickness of the bowel wall is not involved, fistula is uncommon.

**Indications for surgery in Crohn's disease** • Stricture formation, fistula development, and acute intestinal obstruction are recognized complications of Crohn's disease. Failure of response to conservative therapy even without one of these complications may also warrant surgical excision of grossly involved bowel segments. Massive hemorrhage is not generally associated with Crohn's disease.

**Small-bowel fistula** • Small-bowel fistula is a possible complication of any bowel procedure. Postoperative fistulas are, by far, the most common cause. Inflammatory bowel disease, malignancy, and radiation injury are among other, less common, causes. A number of factors predict a low probability of spontaneous fistula closure. These include malignancy, inflammatory bowel disease, distal obstruction, ongoing infection, presence of a foreign body, epithelialization of the fistula tract, and exposed mucosa. Fistulas that close spontaneously do so within 2 months in over 90% of cases. Somatostatin is often used to decrease fistula output but has not been shown to improve the rate or likelihood of spontaneous closure.

**Answers** • 1-D 2-E 3-E 4-C

## CASE PRESENTATION

A 57-year-old man presents to his physician after trace amounts of blood were found in his stool. Colonoscopy is performed and reveals a polyp in his mid transverse colon.

1. Which of the following is a premalignant condition?
   A. Gardner's syndrome
   B. Villous adenoma
   C. Familial polyposis coli
   D. Adenomatous polyp
   E. All of the above
2. The polypoid lesion is excised with a snare through the colonoscope. Pathologic analysis reveals it to be an adenomatous polyp. Carcinoma is identified in the polyp. It is a moderately differentiated tumor with penetration into the muscularis mucosa, but no vascular or lymphatic invasion is seen. There is no malignancy identified in the stalk. Which of these steps is most appropriate?
   A. Subtotal colectomy with primary anastomosis
   B. Transverse colon resection with primary anastomosis
   C. Local excision of the colonic wall surrounding the base of the polyp
   D. Repeat colonoscopy with cautery of the area surrounding the polyp's base
   E. No surgical therapy is indicated in this patient
3. At a subsequent colonoscopic examination, a large sessile polyp is identified in the mid ascending colon. Biopsies reveal a villous adenoma. No evidence of malignancy is seen, although dysplasia is present in the biopsy specimens. Of the following, which would be the most appropriate management of this lesion?
   A. Subtotal colectomy with primary anastomosis
   B. Right hemicolectomy with primary anastomosis
   C. Repeat colonoscopy with cauterization of the remaining lesion
   D. Careful monitoring of the lesion with biopsy every 6 months
   E. No surgical therapy is indicated in this patient
4. What electrolyte abnormality is associated with villous adenoma?
   A. Hypokalemia
   B. Hypernatremia
   C. Hypocalcemia
   D. Hyperphosphatemia
   E. Metabolic alkalosis

## COMMENT

**Malignant potential of colon polyps** • Colon polyps are encountered frequently during screening colonoscopy. When possible, they are resected through the colonoscope. Pathologic identification is important to evaluate the malignant potential of the lesions. Hyperplastic polyps are clearly benign lesions with no malignant potential, but all of those listed in question 1 are premalignant. Adenomatous polyps are less aggressive than the other lesions, but malignancy is found in a small percentage of these lesions. Familial polyposis is an autosomal dominant genetically transmitted disease. Patients have tremendous numbers of adenomatous polyps throughout their colon, with a near-certain likelihood of eventually developing colon carcinoma. Colon resection is generally advocated during early adulthood because the large number of polyps makes screening for development of malignancy difficult, if not impossible. Gardner's syndrome is similar to familial polyposis but is associated with tumors elsewhere in the skin, bone, and subcutaneous tissues. Peutz-Jeghers syndrome is another familial polyposis syndrome characterized by hamartomatous polyps throughout the gastrointestinal tract. These rarely become malignant. Villous adenoma is clearly a premalignant lesion.

**Treatment of malignant polyps** • When malignancy is identified within a colonic polyp, further decision making depends on the depth of invasion and the degree of differentiation. No further therapy is needed after colonoscopic excision of a well-differentiated or moderately differentiated pedunculated polyp in which malignancy is confined to the polyp and the margin of resection is free of tumor. Any invasion into the venous or lymphatic channels necessitates surgical resection even if other prognostic variables are favorable.

**Treatment of sessile polyps** • Premalignant sessile polyps are a more difficult problem. Although some can be safely resected and cauterized piecemeal through the colonoscope, this practice prevents pathologic identification of malignancy in areas destroyed in the process that are not biopsied. In these cases, the safest option is surgical resection.

**Villous adenoma** • As previously noted, villous adenoma is a premalignant lesion that can result in a secretory diarrhea with wasting of potassium.

**Answers** • 1-E 2-E 3-B 4-A

## CASE PRESENTATION

A 54-year-old woman presents to the emergency department with hypotension and melanotic stools. She is resuscitated with fluid and transfused with 4 units of packed red blood cells.

1. Which of the following is least likely to be a cause of her condition?
   A. Colonic diverticulosis
   B. Colonic arteriovenous malformation
   C. Sigmoid diverticulitis
   D. Duodenal ulcer
   E. Ischemic colitis
2. Which of the following would you consider for localizing the source of bleeding?
   A. Angiography
   B. Tagged red blood cell scan
   C. Colonoscopy
   D. Barium enema
   E. A, B, and C
3. Six months later the patient presents to the emergency department with left lower quadrant abdominal pain, fever, and rebound tenderness. Abdominal plain x-rays are unremarkable. Which of the following is the most likely diagnosis?
   A. Sigmoid volvulus
   B. Cecal volvulus
   C. Diverticulosis
   D. Diverticulitis
   E. Sigmoid colon carcinoma
4. An abdominal CT scan performed 6 days later reveals an abscess in the pelvis. The following therapies may be considered; which of them is rarely needed for mild diverticular abscess?
   A. Intravenous maintenance fluid therapy
   B. Intravenous ampicillin/sulbactam (Unasyn)
   C. Maintain patient NPO
   D. Percutaneous drainage of the abscess
   E. Diverting colostomy
5. Which of the following are indications for surgery?
   A. Recurrent episodes of bleeding
   B. Recurrent episodes of inflammation
   C. Chronic stricture formation
   D. Failure to respond to antibiotic therapy
   E. Confirmation of diverticulosis on barium enema examination
   F. A, B, C, and D

## COMMENT

**Causes of massive gastrointestinal tract bleeding** • Melena is an indication of bleeding in the gastrointestinal tract. Massive melena is a life-threatening condition requiring emergent attention. There are numerous possible causes, including diverticulosis, angiodysplasia (arteriovenous malformations), peptic ulcer disease, ulcerative colitis, ischemic colitis, radiation enteritis, variceal hemorrhage, and, particularly in children, Meckel's diverticulum.

**Localization of lower gastrointestinal tract bleeding** • Localization of the site of bleeding is critical should surgical management become necessary. Colonoscopy, angiography, bleeding scan, and upper endoscopy may all help localize the bleeding point. Barium enema is not particularly helpful in this regard unless an obvious abnormality is present, which is unusual.

**Differential diagnosis of diverticulitis** • Diverticulitis is an inflammatory process that originates in pseudodiverticula of the colon. These mucosal pouches occur at weak points in the colon where blood vessels penetrate the bowel wall. The presence of these diverticula can cause massive bleeding. When they become obstructed, inflammation (diverticulitis) can develop. Although it is a dangerous disease in its own right, diverticulitis is not a significant cause of bleeding. Diverticulitis presents with fever and abdominal pain and tenderness localized in the left lower quadrant of the abdomen. Sigmoid and cecal volvulus have characteristic radiographic appearances that distinguish them from diverticulitis. Ischemic colitis is a possible alternative diagnosis and should be considered in patients with a history of complications of atherosclerosis. Colon cancer rarely presents with signs of peritoneal inflammation, and diverticulosis alone is asymptomatic.

**Treatment of diverticular abscess** • Mild episodes of diverticulitis can be treated with oral antibiotic therapy. More severe episodes require inpatient treatment with IV hydration, bowel rest, and IV antibiotic administration. Abscesses may occasionally develop, which can often be treated percutaneously. In the past, treatment often included a proximal diverting colostomy, but this is rarely performed today.

**Indications for surgery** • Indications for resection of colon with diverticula include recurrent episodes of bleeding, particularly if localized to the region of colon most affected (most commonly the sigmoid colon). A single episode of severe diverticulitis may warrant excision, as do recurrent episodes. Recurrent inflammation can also lead to stricture, which may ultimately lead to colonic obstruction if not resected. Failure to respond to antibiotic therapy also warrants excision of the involved bowel. Occasionally, a diverticulum will rupture spontaneously, resulting in diffuse peritonitis. This is a surgical emergency. The presence of diverticulosis by itself is not an indication for surgery. This is a common finding in the elderly patient and is usually asymptomatic. When surgical therapy is required for the acute disease, resection of the involved area is preferred over simple proximal diversion.

**Answers** • 1-C 2-E 3-D 4-E 5-F

## CASE PRESENTATION

A 77-year-old man presents to the emergency department with abdominal distension and crampy abdominal pain. He states that he has not had a bowel movement in the past 72 hours. Abdominal x-ray reveals distended small bowel and a distended colon to the level of the mid descending colon with the rectum measuring 9 cm. in diameter.

1. Which of the following is true?
   - A. Transverse loop colostomy should be performed as soon as possible.
   - B. The radiographic findings suggest that surgical therapy can be delayed and some limited additional evaluation could be performed.
   - C. The presence of small-bowel distension as well as colon distension is more ominous than colon distension alone.
   - D. All of the above.
   - E. A and C.
2. A carcinoma of the mid descending colon is suspected. Necessary additional preoperative evaluation in this patient includes:
   - A. Abdominal CT scan
   - B. CT scan of the chest
   - C. Colonoscopy
   - D. A and C
   - E. None of the above
3. At surgery an obstructing colon cancer is found in the mid descending colon. The tumor has invaded the left kidney and the adjacent abdominal wall. Metastatic lesions are identified throughout the liver, and there is peritoneal tumor studding throughout the abdomen. The most appropriate surgical procedure is:
   - A. Diverting transverse loop colostomy
   - B. Left hemicolectomy with primary colon reanastomosis
   - C. En bloc resection of the left colon, adjacent abdominal wall, and kidney with primary colon reanastomosis
   - D. Left hemicolectomy with end colostomy and mucous fistula formation
   - E. Subtotal colectomy with end ileostomy and Hartmann's pouch
4. Which of the following has been found to be beneficial in patients with this problem?
   - A. Debulking of all visible tumor within the abdomen
   - B. Radiation therapy to the abdominal cavity
   - C. Hepatic artery infusion of chemotherapeutic agents
   - D. All of the above
   - E. None of the above

## COMMENT

**Acute management of large-bowel obstruction** • The patient presents with findings suggestive of complete large-bowel obstruction. Colon perforation with diffuse peritonitis is a serious threat in this condition. The most common site of perforation is the cecum. A cecal diameter greater than 10 cm suggests that perforation is likely imminent and that surgical intervention should not be delayed. In this case, the patient has an incompetent ileocecal valve, allowing for some decompression of the colon into the small bowel. This, and a cecum 9 cm in diameter, suggests that some minimal additional evaluation may be possible. A rectal contrast study may identify the site of obstruction and may also clarify the diagnosis. Colon cancers on the left side of the colon often present with symptoms suggestive of obstruction and have a characteristic "apple core" appearance on contrast studies.

**Management of obstructing colon cancer** • Once the tumor is identified, further workup is not indicated at this time because urgent surgical intervention would be required to relieve the obstruction regardless of the findings. Exploration of the abdomen will be carried out at the time of surgery.

**Surgical management of obstructing colon cancer** • In this case, primary anastomosis would be a poor choice because of the presence of obstruction. Therefore, a colostomy will be required and the patient should be made aware of this preoperatively. The treatment of uncomplicated colon cancer in this location would be a left hemicolectomy. Subtotal colectomy is unnecessary. However, this patient has diffusely metastatic disease and a very poor prognosis. The goal of the procedure is merely to palliate the obstruction caused by the tumor. Extensive and complex resection is not indicated in this setting.

**Treatment of carcinomatosis due to metastatic colon cancer** • Although various systemic chemotherapeutic regimens may be attempted with some chance of tumor remission, tumor debulking, radiation therapy, and hepatic infusion are not indicated.

**Answers** • 1-B 2-E 3-A 4-E

## CASE PRESENTATION

A 65-year-old woman is diagnosed with a carcinoma of the cecum.

1. Of the following, which would be the most likely presenting symptom in this patient?
   A. Small-bowel obstruction
   B. Large-bowel obstruction
   C. Constipation
   D. Anemia
   E. Diarrhea
2. A surgical resection is planned. Preoperative bowel preparation:
   A. Is unnecessary unless there is evidence of obstruction
   B. Is unnecessary for cancers in the right side of the colon
   C. Should be carried out with polyethylene glycol electrolyte solution only
   D. Should include three doses of IV erythromycin
   E. Requires the use of orally administered antibiotic agents
3. The operative procedure of choice is:
   A. Right hemicolectomy with primary ileocolic anastomosis
   B. Right hemicolectomy with end ileostomy and closure of the distal colonic segment
   C. Right hemicolectomy with end ileostomy and mucous fistula formation
   D. Placement of a cecostomy tube
   E. Subtotal colectomy with primary ileorectal anastomosis
4. The pathologic specimen shows a tumor that has invaded through the bowel wall but not into adjacent organs. Three nodes of 14 identified are positive for tumor. There is no evidence of distant metastases. The correct staging for this tumor is:
   A. T1 N2 M1
   B. T2 N1 M0
   C. T3 N2 M1
   D. T3 N1 M0
   E. T4 N0 M0

## COMMENT

**Presentation of colon cancer** • Although it is not always the case, carcinomas of the right colon tend to present with occult blood loss and anemia, whereas carcinomas of the left colon are more likely to present with obstruction than those on the right side.

**Preoperative bowel preparation** • Before elective resection of any of these lesions, a preoperative bowel preparation should be performed to reduce the bacterial count in the colon to lower the risk of postoperative infection. This includes both a mechanical cleansing, most commonly with a polyethylene glycol electrolyte solution, and oral administration of antibiotics that are not absorbed from the GI tract.

**Surgical treatment of colon cancer** • In all colon cancer procedures, the aim of the surgery is to remove the tumor with a margin of uninvolved tissue as well as to remove the lymph nodes draining that area of the colon. There is no advantage in removing the entire colon for a lesion localized in one area. In this case, a right hemicolectomy with primary anastomosis would be the appropriate operation. Primary anastomosis should be avoided in emergent procedures in which an adequate preoperative bowel preparation cannot be performed. In elective resections, however, primary anastomosis is preferred to avoid the complications associated with a subsequent procedure to close the colostomy.

**Tumor staging** • You may argue that this is more detailed information than you will need for the National Board exam (and it will probably not appear on the test); we review it for sake of completeness. The newer TNM classification for colon cancer has replaced the older Duke classification system because it is more precise.

The *T* in this scheme refers to the depth of tumor invasion, in this case T3. The *N* indicates the extent of lymph node involvement, in this case N1 (between one and three nodes involved). The *M* indicates the presence or absence of distant metastases. Because there are no known distant metastatic lesions, this would be an M0 tumor.

**TABLE 1 • The TNM Staging System**

| | |
|---|---|
| **T Levels** | |
| T0 | No evidence of primary tumor |
| TIS | Carcinoma in situ |
| T1 | Tumor invades into submucosa |
| T2 | Tumor invades into muscularis propria |
| T3 | Tumor invades into subserosa or nonperitonealized pericolic or perirectal tissues |
| T4 | Tumor invades through visceral peritoneum or into adjacent organs or structures |
| **N Levels** | |
| N0 | No lymph node involvement |
| N1 | One to three pericolic or perirectal lymph nodes involved |
| N2 | Four or more pericolic or perirectal lymph nodes involved |
| N3 | Metastases to lymph nodes along named vascular trunks |
| **M Levels** | |
| M0 | No distant metastases |
| M1 | Distant metastases present |

**Answers** • 1-D 2-E 3-A 4-D

## CASE PRESENTATION

You are providing care for a 51-year-old man who was recently discharged from the hospital after a T2 N1 M0 cancer of the sigmoid colon was resected. There were no postoperative complications.

1. Appropriate long-term follow up includes:
   A. Carcinoembryonic antigen (CEA) levels every month
   B. Chest x-rays every 3 months for 2 years, then every 6 months
   C. Colonoscopy every 6 months for the next 5 years
   D. Second-look laparotomy 1 year after initial resection
   E. Hepatoiminodiacetic acid (HIDA) scan 6 months following surgery
2. Four years after his initial surgery, a CT scan reveals a mass in the left lobe of his liver. The next step in evaluation of this mass would be:
   A. CEA level
   B. Chest x-ray
   C. Colonoscopy
   D. All of the above
   E. None of the above
3. An isolated metastatic colon cancer lesion is suspected. Which of the following would be the optimal treatment regimen?
   A. Systemic chemotherapy followed by left hepatic lobectomy
   B. Radiation treatment of the involved area of the liver
   C. Hepatic artery infusion of chemotherapeutic agents
   D. Orthotopic liver transplantation
   E. Referral to hospice care

## COMMENT

**Routine screening following colon cancer resection** • After resection of a colon cancer, long-term follow-up is essential. CEA levels should be drawn as a baseline and then followed every 3 to 6 months. Sudden increases should make one suspicious of recurrent tumor. Colonoscopy should be performed about 1 year after surgery and then approximately every 3 years subsequently to evaluate for local tumor recurrence. Chest x-rays are performed fairly frequently at first, with every 3 months being a common practice. After 2 years, the interval may be lengthened, with 6-month intervals being reasonable. Reexploration and HIDA scan have no significant role in follow-up for these tumors.

**Evaluation of liver metastases** • A significant number of patients with isolated liver metastases can be cured of their disease despite this metastatic spread. Preoperative evaluation is aimed at confirming, to the greatest degree possible, that the disease process is, in fact, isolated to one lobe of the liver and that resection will not leave disease behind, either in the liver or elsewhere. (Small lesions in two lobes can be resected, and you don't want to miss the second lesion.) CEA levels will likely be elevated, but extreme elevations may suggest further spread. Colonoscopy should be performed to assess for local tumor recurrence. Chest x-ray will assess for metastatic lung lesions.

**Treatment of isolated liver metastases** • If metastatic disease isolated to a single lobe of the liver is identified, surgical resection is appropriate and may be curative. Preoperative chemotherapy may improve the outcome of this procedure. Hepatic artery infusion of chemotherapeutic agents and radiation therapy have a role in metastatic disease to the liver but should not take the place of resection. Liver transplantation has no role in the treatment of metastatic disease to the liver.

**Answers** • 1-B 2-D 3-A

## CASE PRESENTATION

1. A 25-year-old man complains of finding blood in the toilet after defecation. He has no complaints of pain. Of the following, which is the most likely diagnosis?
   A. Fistula in ano
   B. External hemorrhoids
   C. Perirectal abscess
   D. Internal hemorrhoids
   E. Anal fissure
2. A 31-year-old woman presents with severe unrelenting perianal pain. She has not had a bowel movement since before the pain began. Of the following, which is the most likely?
   A. Fistula in ano
   B. External hemorrhoids
   C. Perirectal abscess
   D. Internal hemorrhoids
   E. Anal fissure
3. A 32-year-old woman presents with complaints of extreme pain with defecation. Of the following, which is the most likely?
   A. Fistula in ano
   B. External hemorrhoids
   C. Perirectal abscess
   D. Internal hemorrhoids
   E. Anal fissure
4. A 32-year-old man presents with a tender area on his left buttock. The area is reddened and seems full but there is no obvious fluctuence or visible purulence. Of the following, which is the most likely?
   A. Fistula in ano
   B. External hemorrhoids
   C. Perirectal abscess
   D. Internal hemorrhoids
   E. Anal fissure
5. One month later the same patient complains of foul-smelling drainage in the perirectal area. On examination, an opening is seen in the left buttock. No other pathology is visible. Of the following, which is the most likely?
   A. Fistula in ano
   B. External hemorrhoids
   C. Perirectal abscess
   D. Internal hemorrhoids
   E. Anal fissure

## COMMENT

**Hemorrhoids** • Perianal disease is a common complaint and often poorly understood. Hemorrhoids represent a spectrum of disease. Often hemorrhoids are divided into "internal" and "external" types. While this is an artificial distinction, it can be useful to describe the symptoms seen in these patients. "Internal hemorrhoids" are contained within the anal canal and often present with bleeding, which on rare occasions can be significant enough to cause anemia. External hemorrhoids are located outside of the anal canal at the anal verge. These are prone to painful episodes of thrombosis. This pain can be severe and is present continuously. Treatment of hemorrhoidal disease is rarely surgical. Conservative therapy is aimed at regulating the bowels to avoid constipation and straining with defecation. The first step is stool softeners and fiber supplements. Indications for operative treatment include pain or bleeding unresponsive to conservative measures.

**Anal fissure** • Pain with defecation usually indicates anal fissure. In this condition, a linear ulcer forms in the anal canal, leading to pain with defecation. The condition is also characterized by periods of remission as the ulcer heals and is then torn open again, often after passage of a particularly large or hard stool. On examination, the fissure is often located posteriorly. A skin tag, referred to as a *sentinel pile,* can often be seen protruding from the anal margin. Conservative measures consist of keeping stools soft and regular with softeners and fiber. If this fails, surgical division of the internal sphincter will decrease pressure in the sphincter and allow healing.

**Perirectal abscess** • Perirectal abscess can cause sepsis if untreated. Like all abscesses, adequate surgical drainage is essential. These abscesses can be difficult to detect by the inexperienced. They are often fairly deep in the perirectal tissues and may not display the same degree of fluctuence and inflammation seen with more superficial infection. These abscesses start in the anal glands located at the dentate line.

**Fistula in ano** • Spontaneous or surgical drainage of a perirectal or perianal abscess can result in formation of a fistulous connection from the anal canal at the dentate line to the external skin. Treatment is surgical and depends on the relationship of the fistula tract to the anal sphincter mechanism.

**Answers** • 1-D 2-B 3-E 4-C 5-A

## CASE PRESENTATION

A 45-year-old woman presents to your office complaining of pain in the right upper quadrant of her abdomen accompanied by mild nausea. The pain is crampy in character and aggravated by fatty foods. It has been present for the past 3 days. She has had no fever and no previous symptoms. On physical examination, she is moderately obese. She has no localized tenderness or rebound tenderness. She is not jaundiced. Gallstones are suspected.

1. Which of the following tests would best confirm this diagnosis?
   A. Abdominal CT scan
   B. Abdominal ultrasound examination
   C. Hepatoiminodiacetic acid (HIDA) scan
   D. Oral cholecystogram
   E. Liver spleen scan
2. Gallstones are, in fact, present in the patient's gallbladder. The common bile duct is normal in size. Which of the following is the most appropriate diagnosis for her pain?
   A. Acute cholecystitis
   B. Chronic cholecystitis
   C. Biliary colic
   D. Cholangitis
   E. Gallstone ileus
3. Cholecystectomy is indicated for which of the following?
   A. Biliary colic
   B. History of gallstone pancreatitis
   C. Ascending cholangitis
   D. Asymptomatic cholelithiasis
   E. A, B, and C
4. A laparoscopic cholecystectomy is performed. Postoperatively, the patient develops jaundice. An ultrasound of the abdomen reveals fluid below the liver in the right upper quadrant. A drain is placed into this fluid collection percutaneously under ultrasound guidance. The most appropriate next step in this patient's management is:
   A. Abdominal CT scan
   B. Return to the operating room for laparoscopic examination of the area
   C. Return to the operating room for exploratory laparotomy
   D. Upper gastrointestinal contrast study
   E. Endoscopic retrograde cholangiopancreatography (ERCP)

## COMMENT

**Identification of gallstones** • Gallstones form when imbalances in the ratios of bile salts, cholesterol, and lecithin in the bile cause crystallization of one or several of these compounds. Ultrasound will identify gallstones better than studies relying on x-ray because most gallstones are radiolucent. HIDA scan may help identify acute cholecystitis because it will demonstrate a failure of gallbladder filling with passage of radioactive marker into the duodenum. The oral cholecystogram has all but been abandoned as a diagnostic test for gallstones. It is prone to false negative and false positive results and is less accurate than other tests.

**Complications of gallstones** • Biliary colic is characterized by crampy abdominal pain caused by the gallbladder contracting against a cystic duct occluded by a stone. Abdominal ultrasound will reveal the presence of gallstones, but other studies are unlikely to be helpful. With cystic duct occlusion, bacterial overgrowth can develop in the gallbladder, resulting in acute cholecystitis. This infection is characterized by peritoneal signs, elevations in white blood cell count, and tenderness in the right upper quadrant of the abdomen. Unlike biliary colic, in which pain is caused by waves of contraction, the pain in acute cholecystitis is more constant and unremitting because the inflammatory process is the cause of the pain rather than peristaltic contractions. Recurrent episodes of inflammation will lead to chronic inflammatory changes in the gallbladder, or chronic cholecystitis. Stone passage into the common bile duct can be occlusive. This will result in jaundice and, if bacterial overgrowth occurs, ascending cholangitis. This life-threatening infection requires some form of drainage of the bile ducts, whether surgical or endoscopic. Gallstone passage through the biliary tree can also cause development of gallstone pancreatitis.

**Indications for surgery in patients with gallstones** • The mere presence of these stones is not, in and of itself, a reason to perform surgery, because many such patients never develop any complications. However, when these stones become symptomatic or a complication develops, gallbladder removal is indicated.

**Complications of laparoscopic cholecystectomy** • Postoperative complications of laparoscopic cholecystectomy, and open cholecystectomy as well, include bile leak and bile duct occlusion. Leaks can occur due to an inadequately ligated cystic duct, a damaged common bile or common hepatic duct, or from unsuspected accessory biliary ducts. Bile duct occlusion is almost always the result of inadvertent ligation of the common bile duct or one of the hepatic ducts. In this case, the fluid collection is drained appropriately. ERCP will identify the site of the leak and may allow for treatment with biliary stents.

**Answers** • 1-B 2-C 3-E 4-E

## CASE PRESENTATION

A 57-year-old man presents with a 3-week history of jaundice. He states that he is experiencing no pain currently but has had occasional abdominal pain over the past several years. He admits to alcohol abuse. He has had no weight loss.

1. Which of the following is true?
   - A. Indirect bilirubin levels rise more than direct bilirubin levels in patients with choledocholithiasis.
   - B. Direct bilirubin elevations are rare in patients with bile duct obstruction proximal to the cystic duct.
   - C. Patients with alcoholic cirrhosis would be expected to have increases in direct bilirubin levels far greater than the increases in indirect bilirubin levels.
   - D. Early primary sclerosing cholangitis is usually associated with elevations in indirect bilirubin levels.
   - E. None of the above.
2. An ultrasound examination reveals areas of intrahepatic bile duct dilatation. The common bile duct could not be well visualized despite a prolonged examination by the ultrasonographer. Of the following, which is the most likely diagnosis?
   - A. Carcinoma of the head of the pancreas
   - B. Carcinoma of the ampulla of Vater
   - C. Sclerosing cholangitis
   - D. Carcinoma of the gallbladder
   - E. All of the above are in the differential diagnosis
3. Endoscopic retrograde cholangiopancreatography reveals profound stenosis of the extrahepatic bile ducts. The intrahepatic ducts have a "beaded" appearance. No malignancy is present. Which of the following is the most definitive treatment for this condition?
   - A. Laparoscopic cholecystectomy
   - B. Long-term steroid therapy
   - C. Choledochoduodenostomy
   - D. Biliary stent placement
   - E. Liver transplant

## COMMENT

**Bilirubin production** • In the liver, unconjugated (indirect) bilirubin is chemically bound to sugars to produce conjugated (direct) bilirubin. The conjugated product is then secreted into the bile. Pathologic processes of the liver tend to inhibit conjugation of bilirubin, leading to increases in indirect bilirubin levels proportionately greater than any increase in direct bilirubin levels. In disease processes leading to obstruction of the biliary tree, levels of direct bilirubin increase (the liver is still able to conjugate bilirubin).

**Differential diagnosis of bile duct obstruction** • Ultrasound may help identify the level of bile duct obstruction. In this case, the lack of a dilated common bile duct makes distal obstruction as occurs in pancreatic and ampullary cancer unlikely. Gallbladder cancer generally does not present with obstructive jaundice. Failure to visualize the common duct with intrahepatic ductal dilatation is, of the alternatives presented, most suggestive of sclerosing cholangitis. Sclerosing bile duct tumors might also give this picture and must always be considered in the differential diagnosis of sclerosing cholangitis.

**Treatment** • The cholangiogram findings described are characteristic of sclerosing cholangitis. There is no cure for this disease; treatments are aimed largely at slowing the disease's progression. Currently, only liver transplant has any hope of assuring long-term relief from this disease.

**Answers** • 1-E 2-C 3-E

## CASE PRESENTATION

A 45-year-old woman comes to the emergency department with a 72-hour history of crampy abdominal pain, frequent vomiting, and nausea. The patient has had neither a bowel movement nor passage of flatus for the past 24 hours. Initial abdominal x-rays reveal multiple loops of air-filled small bowel. There is very little air noted in the colon. In the right upper quadrant of the abdomen, gas is seen within the biliary tract.

1. A set of blood electrolyte levels is drawn. Which of the following statements is true?
   A. Chloride levels are expected to be decreased.
   B. Potassium levels are expected to be low.
   C. Bicarbonate levels are expected to be increased.
   D. Aciduria may be present.
   E. All of the above.
2. Which of the following is true?
   A. The most likely diagnosis is ascending cholangitis.
   B. A complication of gallstones may account for these findings.
   C. Enemas are indicated and should be performed as soon as possible.
   D. Nasogastric decompression and IV fluids will most likely resolve this problem without the need for surgical intervention.
   E. Rapid weight loss over a short time period can cause this clinical picture.
3. At a subsequent procedure, the patient undergoes a cholecystectomy. Pathologic review of the gallbladder reveals an area of carcinoma invading the wall of the gallbladder. Which of the following treatments is appropriate?
   A. Right hepatic lobectomy
   B. Orthotopic liver transplant
   C. Resection of the extrahepatic bile ducts with hepaticojejunostomy reconstruction
   D. Left hepatic lobectomy
   E. Local wedge resection of the liver at the gallbladder fossa with regional lymph node dissection

## COMMENT

**Electrolyte abnormalities in patients with vomiting** • Patients with recurrent episodes of vomiting develop a hypokalemic, hypochloremic, metabolic alkalosis. These patients lose, in their vomitus, significant amounts of chloride and hydrogen ions secreted into the stomach. The resultant dehydration results in renal sodium retention to preserve intravascular volume. Potassium is lost as it is exchanged for sodium in the distal tubule of the nephron under the influence of aldosterone. Despite the metabolic alkalosis, these patients develop a paradoxical aciduria. Chloride depletion leaves only bicarbonate anions to be reabsorbed from the urine along with sodium. Hydrogen ions are excreted into the urine in exchange for sodium ions as the kidneys attempt to hold on to sodium and maintain intravascular volume.

**Gallstone ileus** • Air in the biliary tree along with small-bowel obstruction is characteristic of gallstone ileus. In this condition, a fistula forms between the gallbladder and the duodenum. A large gallstone may then move into the small bowel and cause obstruction, often at the ileocecal valve. Because this is a mechanical obstruction from a foreign body, conservative measures generally will not be effective and surgical treatment is needed. Enemas are not helpful in either treating or diagnosing small-bowel obstruction. Ascending cholangitis is classically associated with right upper quadrant abdominal pain, fever, and jaundice. Rapid weight loss can lead to duodenal obstruction where the superior mesenteric artery (SMA) crosses over the duodenum, trapping it between the SMA and the aorta. This would not lead to diffuse small-bowel dilatation, however, as the obstruction is proximal.

**Gallbladder cancer** • Gallbladder carcinoma is a particularly lethal tumor. Cures generally occur when the tumor is found incidentally at cholecystectomy. For cancer in situ, cholecystectomy is adequate therapy. But in our patient there is invasion of the wall of the gallbladder, and wider resection is needed. The gallbladder fossa is at the junction of the anatomic left and right lobes of the liver. Therefore, single-lobe resection will not obliterate any possible remaining disease. Liver transplant would not be indicated in the face of malignancy. The tumor occurs in the gallbladder and invades into the liver rather than down the biliary tree. Therefore, biliary tree resection is not indicated. Of the choices offered, only local wedge resection with regional lymph node dissection is an option.

**Answers** • 1-E 2-B 3-E

## CASE PRESENTATION

A 44-year-old real estate executive arrives in the emergency department with low blood pressure. He reports "coffee ground" emesis and, on examination, is pale, tachycardic, and diaphoretic.

1. Which of the following statements is true?
   A. Placement of an indwelling urinary catheter should be avoided.
   B. Placement of a nasogastric tube is contraindicated.
   C. Measurement of serum hemoglobin concentration will assess the degree of blood loss.
   D. All of the above.
   E. None of the above.
2. A nasogastric tube is placed and returns bright red blood. Which of the following would be the most appropriate next step in the patient's diagnostic evaluation?
   A. Endoscopic evaluation of the upper GI tract
   B. Immediate laparotomy
   C. Upper gastrointestinal contrast study
   D. Radionuclide bleeding scan
   E. Arteriogram
3. Which of the following conditions is least likely to be associated with massive upper gastrointestinal bleeding?
   A. Peptic ulcer disease
   B. Portal hypertension
   C. Gastric lymphoma
   D. Esophageal rupture (Boerhaave's syndrome)
   E. A, B, and C
   F. All of the above are associated
4. A Mallory-Weiss tear is diagnosed. Which of the following statements is consistent with that diagnosis?
   A. This lesion is usually located on the greater curvature of the stomach.
   B. A history of previous vomiting is not consistent with this diagnosis.
   C. Surgical intervention is infrequently required.
   D. All of the above.
   E. None of the above.

## COMMENT

**Initial management of the patient with upper GI bleeding** • The primary concern for a patient with severe bleeding is restoration of intravascular volume and control of bleeding. Placement of a Foley catheter to monitor urine output is a sensitive marker of intravascular volume status and should be used in any patient with significant bleeding to assure adequate fluid replacement. A nasogastric tube may allow evacuation of blood from the stomach to allow visualization with endoscopy. Hemoglobin levels may drastically underestimate the degree of acute blood loss—hemoglobin and hematocrit may be expected to decline when intravascular volume is replaced.

**Diagnosis of upper GI hemorrhage** • Prior to undertaking any surgical procedure, it is essential to localize the site of bleeding. Endoscopy usually allows precise diagnoses to be made. An arteriogram or bleeding scan may be useful to locate obscure sites of bleeding, but is poor at precise localization. Contrast studies may demonstrate a lesion but do not prove that it is the source of bleeding.

**Differential diagnosis of upper GI bleeding** • The differential diagnosis of massive upper gastrointestinal hemorrhage is long. Possible etiologies include, among others, gastric or duodenal ulcers, Mallory-Weiss tears, gastric tumors, and esophageal varices secondary to portal hypertension. Boerhaave's syndrome is a full-thickness esophageal rupture caused by explosive vomiting. Rather than bleeding, it manifests as mediastinitis and sepsis.

**Mallory-Weiss tear** • This is a partial-thickness tear in the mucosa of the stomach at the gastroesophageal junction usually on the lesser curvature. It occurs with vomiting, and there is a history of vomiting food followed by hematemesis. It usually stops bleeding with conservative measures, and surgical control of hemorrhage is usually not required.

**Answers** • 1-E 2-A 3-E 4-C

## CASE PRESENTATION

A 69-year-old man with anemia is seen by his local physician. Testing of his stool demonstrates the presence of blood.

1. What would be the most appropriate next step in this patient's evaluation?
   A. CT scan of the abdomen
   B. Arteriogram
   C. Radionucleotide bleeding scan
   D. Magnetic resonance imaging (MRI) of the abdomen
   E. Endoscopy of the upper and lower gastrointestinal tracts
2. A gastric ulcer is identified. Which of the following is true?
   A. Benign gastric ulcers are rarely located on the lesser curve of the stomach.
   B. Unlike with duodenal ulcers, *Helicobacter pylori* is rarely associated with benign gastric ulcers.
   C. Gastric ulcers are often associated with low gastric acid production.
   D. Gastric ulcers on the greater curvature of the stomach usually have underlying malignancy.
   E. Ulcers in the body of the stomach are rarely associated with use of nonsteroidal anti-inflammatory agents or aspirin
3. The ulcer is located on the lesser curvature of the stomach. Which of the following would be appropriate initial steps in treating this lesion?
   A. Surgical excision of the ulcer followed by antacid therapy
   B. Endoscopic excision of the ulcer followed by antacid therapy
   C. Antibiotic therapy
   D. Antacid therapy alone
   E. Antacid therapy and antibiotic therapy
4. Which of the following is an indication for surgical treatment of this condition?
   A. Failure to heal after 3 to 6 months of medical therapy
   B. Ulcer recurrence after initial successful nonoperative management
   C. Inability to exclude malignant disease
   D. All of the above
   E. None of the above

## COMMENT

**Evaluation of occult GI blood loss** • There are many possible causes for occult GI blood loss. Most can be diagnosed with endoscopy, which also allows biopsy and, in some cases, therapy (i.e., polyp excision). Arteriogram may be useful to localize and control acute massive bleeding but cannot demonstrate a "slow leak." The same is true of the radionuclide bleeding scan. CT scan and MRI will not identify small lesions such as peptic ulcer disease or colonic polyps.

**Pathophysiology of gastric ulcers** • Benign gastric ulcers are most commonly found on the lesser curvature of the stomach and are very commonly associated with *Helicobacter pylori*. Ulcers elsewhere in the stomach are rare but do occur and are often associated with use of nonsteroidal anti-inflammatory agents. Any gastric ulcer can be the result of an underlying malignancy. Ulcers located away from the lesser curvature have no higher incidence of malignancy than ulcers located along the lesser curvature. Many, although not all, types of benign gastric ulcers are associated with low gastric acid secretion rates, unlike duodenal or prepyloric ulcers, where increased acidity is the norm.

**Treatment** • The initial treatment of a gastric ulcer not associated with massive bleeding or perforation is medical. Treatment consists of antacid therapy even in those cases where there is low acid production. *H. pylori* is very often present in these patients, so antibiotic therapy aimed at *H. pylori* is an important component of treatment.

**Indications for surgery in gastric ulcer** • Indications for surgery include acute complications such as perforation or hemorrhage as well as inability to exclude malignancy. Failure to heal despite maximal medical therapy and recurrence of the ulcer after therapy would also be indications for surgical intervention.

**Answers** • 1-E 2-C 3-E 4-D

## CASE PRESENTATION

A short, 35-year-old woman weighing 340 pounds seeks surgical correction. She has tried several weight loss plans under the supervision of her family physician but has been unable to sustain significant weight loss. She has developed hypertension and poorly controlled diabetes.

1. Indications for surgical therapy for obesity include:
   A. Body mass index of 38 kg/m$^2$ and sleep apnea
   B. Body mass index of 37 kg/m$^2$, hypertension, and diabetes
   C. Body mass index of 42 kg/m$^2$ and degenerative joint disease
   D. All of the above
2. The patient undergoes a Roux-en-Y gastric bypass procedure. Long-term complications include which of the following:
   A. Iron deficiency anemia
   B. Calcium deficiency
   C. $B_{12}$ deficiency
   D. Gallstones
   E. Hypoglycemia
   F. A, B, C, and D
3. Long-term requirements for this patient include:
   A. Daily vitamin supplements
   B. Ursodiol (Actigall)
   C. Calcium tablet daily
   D. All of the above
   E. None of the above

## COMMENT

**Indications for surgery in the morbidly obese** • Surgical therapy has been proven to be beneficial in patients with morbid obesity. However, the complication rate is high, requiring careful patient selection. Body mass index (BMI) is a useful and widely accepted measure of the degree of obesity. This is calculated by dividing the patient's weight in kilograms by the square of the patient's height in meters. Patients with a BMI greater than 40 kg/m$^2$ are considered morbidly obese and warrant consideration for surgical therapy based on BMI alone. For those with obesity-related complications such as hypertension, diabetes, degenerative joint disease, and sleep apnea, surgical therapy may also be appropriate even with a BMI as low as 35 kg/m$^2$.

**Long-term complications of obesity surgery** • Operative procedures for obesity have significant long-term nutritional sequelae. Jejunoileal bypass creates a short-bowel syndrome limiting nutrient absorption but has been largely abandoned because of severe long-term complications, including lethal hepatic failure. Various gastric restrictive procedures are now employed, with the Roux-en-Y gastric bypass the current favorite. Nutritional complications do occur and require ongoing monitoring. Iron deficiency and calcium deficiency result from bypass of normal nutrient flow through the duodenum and proximal jejunum. Calcium and iron are largely absorbed in these areas that are bypassed by the gastric bypass procedure. Decreasing the gastric reservoir diminishes the release of intrinsic factor, impairing absorption of vitamin $B_{12}$. Gallstones also occur and are most commonly a problem during the rapid weight loss phase within the first several months of surgery.

**Long-term requirements after obesity surgery** • Because of the problems described above, patients need multivitamins, calcium, and oral vitamin $B_{12}$. Actigall is used during the first 6 months following surgery to minimize the formation of gallstones.

**Answers** • 1-D 2-F 3-D

## CASE PRESENTATION

A previously healthy 44-year-old mutual fund manager presents with acute onset of severe abdominal pain. The pain started in the epigastrium but is now located diffusely throughout the abdomen. On physical examination, his abdomen is rigid and bowel sounds are diminished. On x-ray, air is noted under the diaphragm.

1. Which of the following would be the most appropriate next step?
   A. Upper gastrointestinal endoscopy
   B. Upper gastrointestinal contrast study
   C. CT scan of the abdomen
   D. Exploratory laparotomy
   E. Hepatoiminodiacetic acid (HIDA) scan
2. After initial evaluation he has surgery, during which a perforated duodenal ulcer is identified. Which of the following is true about the operative procedures available for treatment of this condition?
   A. Truncal vagotomy with antrectomy is less likely to result in diarrhea than other procedures.
   B. Highly selective vagotomy has a high incidence of postoperative "dumping syndrome."
   C. Simple patching of the ulcer with omentum is adequate surgical therapy.
   D. Treatment for *Helicobacter pylori* is necessary after highly selective vagotomy but not after truncal vagotomy.
   E. All of the above are true.
3. Six months after truncal vagotomy and gastric antrectomy with oversewing of the proximal duodenum and gastrojejunostomy (Billroth II procedure), the patient presents with complaints of abdominal pain relieved by vomiting. The vomitus is bilious in nature with few food particles. Which of the following is the most likely diagnosis?
   A. Afferent limb obstruction
   B. Postoperative pancreatitis
   C. Dumping syndrome
   D. Stenosis of the gastrojejunal anastomosis
   E. Ulceration of the jejunum at the gastrojejunostomy (stomal ulcer)

## COMMENT

**Treatment for perforated viscus** • In the absence of recent surgery or invasive procedures, the presence of air outside of the gastrointestinal tract in the abdomen indicates that some air-containing structure within the abdomen (i.e., bowel) has perforated. No further diagnostic testing is indicated because, regardless of the results, surgery will be required. The exact location of the perforation will be found at surgery.

**Surgical procedures for peptic ulcer disease** • A number of operations have been developed for acid reduction in the treatment of peptic ulcer disease. Unfortunately, the more effective the procedure is at reducing the rate of ulcer recurrence, the more likely the development of significantly disabling complications. Any procedure involving division of the main trunk of the vagus nerve can lead to problems with diarrhea. Thus, vagotomy and pyloroplasty, vagotomy and gastrojejunostomy, vagotomy and antrectomy, and vagotomy and subtotal gastrectomy all can lead to chronic diarrhea. Dumping syndrome is characterized by abdominal discomfort, tachycardia, faintness, sweating, and diarrhea associated with food intake. Highly selective vagotomy has a lower incidence of dumping syndrome and diarrhea. It is, however, technically more demanding than other procedures and in some series has an unacceptably high ulcer recurrence rate. In patients with no previous history of peptic ulcer disease or in unstable patients, simple patching of the perforation with omentum is preferred. It is also becoming more apparent that, with the recognition of *H. pylori* as a causative agent in many, if not most, ulcers, lesser operative procedures can now be performed with acceptable recurrence rates. Many patients with peptic ulcer disease are colonized with *H. pylori,* and treatment for this organism is indicated regardless of the procedure performed.

**Other complications of ulcer surgery** • As stated previously, more complex operative procedures for treating peptic ulcer disease are associated with a number of significant complications. This patient shows classic signs of afferent limb obstruction (afferent loop syndrome). In this condition, the segment of bowel between the duodenal stump and the gastrojejunostomy becomes partially obstructed and distended with fluids produced by the liver and pancreas. This distension causes pain. As the pressure builds in the afferent limb, the obstruction is suddenly relieved with relief of pain and vomiting of the bilious contents of the previously obstructed afferent limb.

Alkaline reflux gastritis occurs when bile and pancreatic secretions from the afferent limb bathe the stomach at the gastrojejunostomy. The pain of this condition is not relieved by vomiting. Stomal ulcerations and strictures of the gastrojejunostomy may also occur and present with pain and obstruction, respectively. Pancreatitis is not a complication of ulcer surgery, and pancreatitis causes unrelenting pain.

**Answers** • 1-D 2-C 3-A

## CASE PRESENTATION

A 44-year-old general surgeon complains of nocturnal heartburn associated with regurgitation into the back of his throat. He also has occasional episodes of spasmodic retrosternal chest pain. Proton pump inhibitors and other medical therapies have been tried with little symptomatic relief.

1. The most important study to document gastroesophageal acid reflux is:
   A. Endoscopy
   B. Barium swallow
   C. Esophageal manometry
   D. pH probe
   E. Radionuclide gastric emptying study
2. Severe gastroesophageal acid reflux is documented. The next step in the patient's treatment plan is:
   A. Laparoscopic Nissen fundoplication
   B. Distal esophagectomy
   C. Esophagoscopy with biopsy of gastroesophageal junction
   D. Truncal vagotomy and gastric antrectomy
   E. Barium swallow
3. After an appropriate evaluation, a laparoscopic Nissen fundoplication is performed. Two weeks later, after a bout of vomiting, the patient develops food intolerance and chest pain. He states that he feels "bloated." The diagnostic test most likely to reveal the diagnosis is:
   A. Esophagoscopy
   B. CT scan of the abdomen
   C. Ultrasound of the right upper quadrant of the abdomen
   D. Barium swallow
   E. Endoscopic ultrasound study of the gastroesophageal junction

## COMMENT

**Diagnosis of gastroesophageal reflux** • Diagnosis of gastroesophageal (GE) reflux is dependent on documenting acid reflux into the esophagus. This is most accurately accomplished with a pH probe study. Contrast swallow is able to identify the presence of a hiatal hernia but demonstrates GE reflux in less than half of patients who ultimately prove to have the disease. The presence of a hiatal hernia, by itself, does not imply significant GE reflux, nor does it alone warrant surgical repair. Manometry is used to diagnose disease affecting peristalsis in the esophagus and alterations in the pressure of the lower esophageal sphincter. It does not, however, document reflux. Endoscopy may detect the presence of esophagitis but does not definitively document the presence of acid reflux into the esophagus.

**Preoperative evaluation** • Prior to operative intervention, it is imperative to document that Barrett's esophagus is not present. This requires endoscopy with biopsy of any area of esophagitis. In some cases, manometry may also be indicated to rule out functional disorders of the esophagus. These could cause severe problems if a reflux operation is performed to increase pressure at the GE junction in the presence of aperistalsis, as occurs in achalasia.

**Postoperative complications** • The symptoms described are typical for movement of the "gastric wrap" performed in a fundoplication through the esophageal hiatus and into the chest. This typically occurs with vomiting and may result from failure to adequately plicate the esophageal hiatus at the time of surgery. Barium swallow demonstrates the abnormality.

**Answers** • 1-D 2-C 3-D

## CASE PRESENTATION

A 40-year-old man received a cadaveric kidney transplant 2 years earlier. His medical history includes hypertension and type II diabetes. He is currently taking cyclosporine, mycophenolate mofetil (CellCept), and prednisone for immunosuppression, with a stable baseline creatinine level of 1.5. Four days ago he was seen in a local emergency room with low-grade fever and productive cough. Chest x-ray showed a small right lower lobe infiltrate. Clarithromycin was prescribed for community-acquired pneumonia. He now presents to your office complaining of increased shortness of breath and swelling. The chest x-ray now shows a dense and large lobar infiltrate on the right side. $O_2$ saturation is 90% on room air. Serum creatinine level is 7.0.

1. What is going on with this patient?
   A. Worsening pneumonia
   B. Dehydration
   C. Cyclosporine toxicity
   D. Rejection of the transplant kidney
   E. A and C
2. If the patient has worsening pneumonia, what would be the appropriate course of treatment?
   A. Start IV antibiotics and continue current immunosuppression.
   B. Start IV antibiotics, continue prednisone and cyclosporine, and stop mycophenolate mofetil.
   C. Start IV antibiotics, continue cyclosporine, and stop prednisone and mycophenolate mofetil.
   D. Start IV antibiotics and stop all immunosuppression.
3. Which of the following is a side effect of cyclosporine toxicity?
   A. Hyperkalemia
   B. Hypertension
   C. Neurotoxicity
   D. Hirsutism
   E. All of the above

## COMMENT

**Immune suppression agents in the transplant patient** • Since the introduction of cyclosporine in the early 1980s, kidney transplant has become an accepted treatment of end-stage renal disease. Currently, the 1-year patient survival is 97% and graft survival is 90% to 92%. The most common immunosuppressive agents include cyclosporine or FK506 (Prograf), prednisone, and mycophenolate mofetil (CellCept) or sirolimus (rapamycin). Cyclosporine and FK506 are calcineurin inhibitors that lead to decreased interleukin-2 production. Their metabolism is cytochrome P-450 dependent. Therefore, medications that affect the cytochrome P-450 system will affect the cyclosporine and FK506 level. Macrolide antibiotics (erythromycin, clarithromycin, josamycin, but not azithromycin), azole antifungals (fluconazole, itraconazole, ketoconazole), and calcium channel blockers (diltiazem, verapamil, nicardipine, but not nifedipine, felodipine) are commonly prescribed medications that can increase cyclosporine level and cause toxicity. Cyclosporine toxicity resulted in acute renal failure in this patient. This patient's clinical history is consistent with acute renal failure from nephrotoxicity secondary to elevated cyclosporine level.

**Treatment of infection in the transplant patient** • When the patient presents with minor infection, change in immunosuppression medication is not needed. With moderate infection, mycophenolate mofetil and rapamycin should be held. Immunosuppression should be stopped completely if the patient has a life-threatening infection.

**Side effects of cyclosporine** • Some of the common toxicity side effects of cyclosporine include neurotoxicity, nephrotoxicity, hypertension, hyperkalemia, hypercholesterolemia, hirsutism, gingival hyperplasia, and hypomagnesemia. Treatment includes checking a cyclosporine level to confirm the diagnosis, holding cyclosporine until the level is down, dialysis as needed, and supportive care.

**Answers** • 1-E 2-D 3-E

## CASE PRESENTATION

A 62-year-old man is scheduled to have an exploratory laparotomy for possible colon cancer. The patient weighs 70 kg. The anesthesia for the procedure will consist of general anesthesia and epidural analgesia.

1. The epidural catheter is inserted and 15 cc of 2% Xylocaine is administered via the epidural catheter. Signs of an intravascular injection include:
   A. Tinnitus and dizziness and blurred vision
   B. Pruritus
   C. Seizures
   D. All of the above
   E. A and C
2. After general anesthesia is induced with sodium thiopental, succinylcholine is administered for paralysis. Contraindications to succinylcholine include:
   A. Spinal cord injury with quadriplegia
   B. Hyperkalemia
   C. Recent third-degree burn covering 40% of total body surface area
   D. Family history of malignant hyperthermia
   E. All of the above
3. Throughout the case, general anesthesia is maintained with isoflurane and nitrous oxide. Thirty minutes after general anesthesia is induced, the patient's heart rate is 130 and his temperature is 39°C. Malignant hyperthermia is characterized by:
   A. Respiratory acidosis
   B. Skeletal muscle rigidity and rhabdomyolysis
   C. Metabolic acidosis
   D. All of the above
   E. A and C

## COMMENT

**Complications of local anesthetic agents** • Local anesthetic toxicity usually results from accidental intravascular injection or increased uptake from the perivascular space. The toxicity of local anesthetics is dose dependent. Signs and symptoms of local anesthetic toxicity in order of increasing plasma concentrations include circumoral numbness, tongue paresthesia, dizziness, visual and auditory disturbances, seizures, coma, respiratory arrest, and cardiovascular depression.

**Contraindications to use of depolarizing agents** • Succinylcholine is a depolarizing muscle relaxant that resembles acetylcholine, acts at the postjunctional neuromuscular membrane, and usually produces muscle fasciculations. Succinylcholine is a known triggering agent of malignant hyperthermia and should be avoided in all patients with a known susceptibility or family history of malignant hyperthermia. Succinylcholine is contraindicated in patients with spinal cord injury, burn injury, myopathies, and stroke because it can cause life-threatening elevations in potassium levels.

**Malignant hyperthermia** • Malignant hyperthermia (MH) is a disease of abnormal calcium release from the sarcoplasmic reticulum that results in tachypnea, metabolic acidosis, respiratory acidosis, skeletal muscle rigidity, tachycardia, hypertension, rhabdomyolysis, and increased plasma levels of potassium, calcium, and lactate. Triggers for MH include depolarizing muscle relaxants and all potent volatile anesthetics. Safe anesthetic agents include nitrous oxide, propofol, all local anesthetics, and all nondepolarizing muscle relaxants. The disease shows an autosomal dominant pattern of inheritance with variable expression. Treatment of MH includes rapid elimination of all triggering agents, aggressive ventilation, cooling if fever is present, and administration of dantrolene. Dantrolene inhibits calcium release from the sarcoplasmic reticulum and is used in treatment as well as prevention in MH-susceptible patients.

**Answers** • 1-E 2-E 3-D

## CASE PRESENTATION

A 56-year-old man is scheduled for a left knee arthroscopy. He weighs 85 kg.

1. Prior to surgery, the patient is complaining of severe knee pain. Which of the following will help relieve his pain?
   A. Morphine and oxycodone
   B. Fentanyl
   C. Ketorolac
   D. Midazolam or diazepam
   E. A, B, and C
2. Prior to inducing anesthesia, the patient tells you that he ate a hamburger, fries, and a small drink just 2 hours ago. You should:
   A. Continue with the surgery as scheduled without delay
   B. Administer metoclopramide, cimetidine, and sodium bicitrate, then proceed without delay
   C. Delay the case for 6 to 8 hours from the time of the meal
   D. Insert a nasogastric tube, suction out the gastric contents, and then proceed without delay
   E. None of the above
3. On postoperative day 3 the patient has fever and elevated levels of AST and ALT. Which of the following drugs may be responsible?
   A. Halothane
   B. Succinylcholine
   C. Sodium thiopental
   D. Morphine
   E. Midazolam

## COMMENT

**Pain relief** • Drugs commonly used for their analgesic properties include opioids and nonsteroidal anti-inflammatory drugs (NSAIDs). Opioids such as morphine, meperidine, fentanyl, oxycodone, and hydromorphone provide analgesia by occupying the μ-1 and μ-2 receptors, thus inhibiting nociceptive neuron neurotransmitter release. NSAIDs provide analgesia by interfering with prostaglandin synthesis. Benzodiazepines such as midazolam and diazepam provide sedation and amnesia but not analgesia.

**Preoperative management** • Except for specially instructed medications, patients scheduled for elective surgery should not take anything by mouth for 8 hours preceding the surgery. Patients who are at increased risk for aspiration, such as those with a hiatal hernia or gastroesophageal reflux disease, may receive preoperative medications to decrease the volume and acidity of gastric contents. These drugs include histamine-2 blockers such as cimetidine, clear liquid antacids such as magnesium citrate, and gastrointestinal promotility agents such as metoclopramide. In these high-risk patients or in those requiring intubation without an appropriate preoperative period of fasting, general anesthesia may be induced via rapid sequence induction. This technique consists of maintaining manually applied external cricoid pressure until correct placement of a cuffed endotracheal tube is confirmed.

**Anesthesia-related hepatitis** • The common causes of postoperative hepatic dysfunction include viral hepatitis, impaired hepatic perfusion, hepatocyte hypoxia, sepsis, hemolysis, sepsis, and drug-induced hepatitis. Halothane hepatitis is extremely rare (1 per 35,000 cases), and it may lead to hepatic necrosis and death. Typically, hepatic dysfunction is manifested as fever and elevated aminotransferases within the first postoperative week. Risk factors for halothane hepatitis include repeat administration of halothane within 4 weeks of a previous halothane anesthetic, middle-aged obese women, and persons with a familial predisposition to halothane toxicity. Halothane hepatitis primarily affects adults and children past puberty. For these reasons, halothane is not commonly used as an anesthetic agent currently.

**Answers** • 1-E 2-C 3-A

## CASE PRESENTATION

A 43-year-old right-hand-dominant woman presents to your office complaining of a 2-month history of worsening pain, numbness, and tingling in her right thumb, index finger, and long finger. She has had no treatment to date but she thinks that she has carpal tunnel syndrome.

1. Which of the following statements about carpal tunnel syndrome is true?
   A. It is more common in males than in females.
   B. It is unilateral in most cases.
   C. Pregnant patients may have spontaneous improvement in symptoms after delivery.
   D. The average age of patients with carpal tunnel syndrome is approximately 30 years.
   E. All of the above.
2. Which clinical finding is most characteristic of moderate carpal tunnel syndrome?
   A. Pain awakens patient from sleep frequently and gets better during the day.
   B. Pain is worst during the day and gets better at night or at rest.
   C. Numbness is worst during the day when the hands are at rest.
   D. Frequent dropping of items such as coffee cups from hands.
   E. Shaking of the hand worsens symptoms.
3. Which physical finding is most characteristic of carpal tunnel syndrome?
   A. Positive Phalen's sign (increased numbness with wrist flexion)
   B. Positive Finkelstein's test (pain in distal radial forearm with ulnar wrist deviation)
   C. Negative Tinel's test at the carpal tunnel (failure to elicit an "electric shock" sensation with percussion over the carpal tunnel)
   D. Abnormal two-point discrimination (inability to separately distinguish touch at two points separated by 15 mm)
   E. All of the above are characteristic of carpal tunnel syndrome
4. If, by clinical exam and electrodiagnostic studies, our patient is found to have moderate carpal tunnel syndrome, what would be the next step in treatment?
   A. Injection of Celestone into the carpal tunnel.
   B. A wrist cock-up splint and perform an ergonomic check of work environment
   C. Open carpal tunnel release
   D. A short arm thumb spica splint and take nonsteroidal anti-inflammatory agents by mouth
   E. Narcotic pain relievers at bedtime

## COMMENT

**Carpal tunnel syndrome** • Carpal tunnel syndrome is caused by a compression of the median nerve at the carpal tunnel. Seventy percent of patients are female, and the average age of diagnosis is 54 years. It is bilateral in 60% of patients. Most cases are idiopathic, but thyroid disorders, pregnancy, diabetes, arthritis, and tumors in the carpal tunnel can cause or aggravate the syndrome. Many cases of pregnancy-aggravated carpal tunnel syndrome will spontaneously subside after delivery.

**History findings characteristic of carpal tunnel syndrome** • Classically, the presentation is of pain, numbness, and tingling of the thumb, index, and long fingers (the sensory distribution of the median nerve in the hand). It is typically worse at night and is accompanied very often by nocturnal awakening. Patients often state that shaking the hand helps. It usually gets better during the day, but activities that require wrist flexion and gripping, such as holding a coffee cup or driving with hands on top of the steering wheel, often make it worse. Dropping items from hands is a characteristic of severe carpal tunnel syndrome and is due to damage to the motor branch of the median nerve at the carpal tunnel, which is a late finding.

**Physical examination** • Compression of the median nerve at the carpal tunnel results in nerve dysfunction. Effective tests include Phalen's test, carpal compression test, Tinel's test, and two-point discrimination testing. *Phalen's test* is performed by flexing the wrists firmly with the arms otherwise held in a relaxed position. Increased numbness within 1 minute indicates a positive test. The *carpal compression test* is performed by compressing the volar side of the wrist firmly with an examining finger. Increased numbness within 1 minute indicates a positive test. *Tinel's test* is performed at the carpal tunnel by percussing the volar side of the wrist with an examining finger. In patients with carpal tunnel syndrome, an "electric shock" will be felt in the distribution of the median nerve in the hand. A *two-point discrimination test* is performed by lightly touching two thin wires, separated by a specified distance, to the fingertip. Normally, correctly discerning two points occurs at 5 mm of separation (10 mm in patients with calluses). A measurement of greater than 15 mm is abnormal and indicates a decrease in nerve function. Two-point discrimination is less sensitive for carpal tunnel syndrome than a Phalen's test and will be abnormal in peripheral neuropathy of any etiology. Other etiologies, such as diabetes, should be considered. *Finkelstein's test* is performed by placing the thumb into a closed fist and ulnarly deviating the wrist. A positive test, indicated by pain on the distal radial forearm, is classic in de Quervain's tenosynovitis of the first dorsal compartment. Pain can also be elicited with this maneuver in patients with osteoarthritis of the first carpometacarpal joint, which is common.

**Treatment** • Initial therapy of mild and moderate carpal tunnel syndrome should be a wrist cock-up splint (worn especially at night) and ergonomic changes at work (wrist-neutralizing props and good posture). The use of NSAIDs may help as well. Further therapy may include steroid injections that often relieve pain for 3 to 5 weeks. This can be used as a diagnostic trial as well. Definitive therapy is by open or endoscopic carpal tunnel release. In the case of an electromyogram that indicates fibrillations of the abductor pollicis muscle, an urgent carpal tunnel release is indicated without further nonoperative treatment.

**Answers** • 1-C 2-A 3-A 4-B

## CASE PRESENTATION

A 34-year-old right-hand-dominant man presents with a 3-day history of progressively worsening pain and swelling around his left small fingernail. There has been no drainage from the site and there is no tracking cellulitis identified. He denies any history of trauma to the area and is in good health, except for diabetes. You diagnosis a paronychia.

1. What is the most likely causative organism?
   A. *Candida albicans*
   B. *Staphylococcus aureus*
   C. *Mycobacterium marinum*
   D. *Pseudomonas aeruginosa*
   E. *Escherichia coli*
2. What treatment is indicated?
   A. An oral cephalosporin for 1 week
   B. An oral antifungal agent for 6 weeks
   C. Removal of all or part of the nail plate and an oral cephalosporin for 1 week
   D. Intravenous penicillin for 5 days
   E. Warm soaks until the infection "points," then incision and drainage
3. The patient refuses treatment but returns 4 days later with swelling on the volar fingertip pad in addition to around the nail. What is the most likely new diagnosis?
   A. Felon
   B. Paronychia
   C. Necrotizing fasciitis
   D. Flexor tenosynovitis
   E. Osteomyelitis
4. What additional treatment is indicated now?
   A. An oral cephalosporin for 2 weeks
   B. Incision and drainage of the pulp of the fingertip and an oral cephalosporin for 1 week
   C. Incision and drainage of the pulp of the fingertip and an intravenous cephalosporin for 2 weeks
   D. Hyperbaric oxygen therapy
   E. Insertion of a long-term venous access catheter and 6 weeks of intravenous cephalosporin therapy

## COMMENT

**Causative organisms in acute paronychia** • This common infection occurs very often without antecedent trauma. The most common causative agent is *S. aureus*. *C. albicans* is the most common causative agent in chronic paronychia, not acute paronychia. *M. marinum* infections typically occur after exposure to seawater or aquariums. The other organisms mentioned are not commonly associated with fingertip infections.

**Treatment of paronychia** • The treatment for all but the earliest paronychias is removal of the nail plate associated with the infection followed with oral antibiotics that cover Gram-positive organisms. The removal of the nail plate effectively drains the abscess and allows proper regrowth of the nail without deformity.

**Felon** • After refusing appropriate therapy, the patient returns several days later with an extension of the paronychia infection into the volar fingertip pad. A felon, as this infection is called, is very painful and can be caused by extension of an untreated or poorly treated paronychia or by direct trauma to the fingertip.

**Treatment of a felon** • The best treatment now is clearly incision and drainage followed by oral antibiotics. The fingertip has multiple longitudinal fibrous septa that compartmentalize the infection initially. As pressure in a compartment grows, perforation into an adjacent compartment occurs. Drainage of the abscess requires complete release of all involved compartments. A mid-lateral incision is often used for this procedure. If all compartments are not fully drained, the felon will persist, possibly even infecting the flexor tendon sheath.

**Answers** • 1-B 2-C 3-A 4-B

## CASE PRESENTATION

A 21-year-old man presents with a swollen, tender, right fourth metacarpophalangeal joint. On examination, there is a 3-mm laceration over the joint. The area around the joint is erythematous, swollen, and tender. He states that he was involved in a fight the previous afternoon and sustained the cut sometime during the fight.

1. Which of the following statements about tetanus prophylaxis is true?
   - A. This patient's wound would not be considered tetanus prone.
   - B. Tetanus immune globulin is never indicated for wounds felt *not* to be tetanus prone.
   - C. Tetanus immune globulin is always necessary in wounds considered tetanus prone.
   - D. A patient with a tetanus-prone wound who has been completely immunized and whose last booster was 9 years ago requires neither tetanus immune globulin nor tetanus toxoid.
   - E. All of the above are true.
2. What other treatment is indicated?
   - A. An oral cephalosporin for 1 week
   - B. IV cephalosporin for 1 week
   - C. Hyperbaric oxygen therapy
   - D. Emergent exploration of the joint
   - E. Warm soaks, hand elevation, and oral penicillin G
3. A year later, after sustaining a minor laceration at work, the patient returns complaining of severe pain along the volar aspect of the entire finger, extending into the palm. Attempted flexion of the involved finger causes severe pain. What treatment is indicated now?
   - A. Warm soaks, elevation, and oral cephalosporin therapy
   - B. Warm soaks, elevation, and IV cephalosporin therapy
   - C. Incision and drainage of the flexor tendon sheath with IV antibiotic therapy
   - D. Hyperbaric oxygen therapy
   - E. Warm soaks and elevation alone

## COMMENT

**Tetanus prophylaxis** • Any patient with a significant open wound should be considered for tetanus prophylaxis with tetanus toxoid and possibly tetanus immune globulin as well. Tetanus-prone wounds include wounds more than 6 hours old, complex lacerations, wounds greater than 1 cm in depth, and wounds with devitalized tissue, contamination, or signs of infection. Burn wounds, crush injuries, projectile wounds, and frostbite wounds should also be considered tetanus prone. A history of complete immunization is important, as well as the time since the patient's last booster. In wounds not considered tetanus prone, tetanus immune globulin is not indicated regardless of previous immunization status. It should be given, however, to any patient with a tetanus-prone wound who has not been completely immunized (at least 3 previous doses and less than 10 years since the last booster).

Tetanus toxoid (available combined with diphtheria toxoid) should be given to any patient without complete immunization regardless of whether the wound is tetanus prone or not. It is indicated in completely immunized patients only if it has been more than 10 years since the last booster for non-tetanus-prone wounds or less than 5 years for tetanus-prone wounds.

**"Fight bites"** • Infection in the metacarpophalangeal joints with a laceration nearby, especially on the dominant hand, are almost always caused by human tooth penetration during a fight. A careful history is essential because patients will often deny that they were involved in a fight. Emergent exploration of the joint with irrigation and drainage followed by antibiotics to cover both *Staphylococcus aureus* (most common) and *Eikenella corrodens* (also frequently found) is essential. Often, fragments of teeth are found imbedded in the cartilage and must be removed along with any damaged cartilage.

Hyperbaric oxygen treatment involves exposure of the patient to high levels of oxygen. This raises oxygen tension in wounds and can be effective in chronic wounds such as osteoradionecrosis of the mandible but is not indicated in acute infections such as this. It also is not indicated until incision and drainage of pus and debridement of devitalized tissues have been accomplished.

**Flexor tenosynovitis** • Flexor tenosynovitis is an infection of the tendon sheath. Penetrating trauma is the most common etiology for this infection, but extension from a felon occurs frequently as well. Again, *S. aureus* is the most common bacteria cultured. This is a serious infection that requires emergent incision and drainage as well as intravenous antibiotics. Classically, there are four signs of flexor tenosynovitis: flexed posture of the finger, fusiform swelling, tenderness of the flexor tendon sheath, and pain on passive stretch of the finger. These are known as Kanavel's signs.

Failure to treat any infection of the hand or fingers promptly and effectively will result in progression of the infection, worsening of functional outcome, and even amputation of a finger or a hand.

**Answers** • 1-B 2-D 3-C

## CASE PRESENTATION

A 47-year-old woman with no family history of breast cancer is diagnosed with invasive ductal carcinoma. The mass in her right breast comprises 50% of the total volume of the breast. Her surgeon recommends a mastectomy with sentinel lymph node biopsy.

1. Which of the following statements is true?
   A. Immediate reconstruction is always contraindicated in patients with invasive ductal carcinoma of the breast.
   B. Breast reconstruction cannot be accomplished in patients undergoing mastectomy unless the axilla is left undisturbed.
   C. Reconstruction should be delayed for 5 years in patients with documented malignancy to ensure that the patient is disease free before proceeding.
   D. Immediate reconstruction should not be attempted in patients with invasive ductal carcinoma unless the tumor is smaller than 2 cm in diameter.
   E. The final outcome, aesthetically, will be better with mastectomy and immediate reconstruction than with lumpectomy in this case.
2. What is the best timing of breast reconstruction surgery after mastectomy?
   A. Reconstruction should be delayed for 6 weeks after all chemotherapy and radiation therapy has been given.
   B. Immediate breast reconstruction is contraindicated in patients who will require radiation therapy, but not those requiring chemotherapy.
   C. If reconstruction is done at the time of mastectomy, radiation therapy and chemotherapy should be delayed for 2 weeks.
   D. All of the above are true.
   E. A and C are true.
3. Which of the following is the most common complication of reconstruction with an implant?
   A. Capsular contracture
   B. Infection
   C. Scar tissue that feels like recurrent cancer
   D. Bleeding
   E. Autoimmune disorders
4. Which of the complications of reconstruction with implants is avoided by a TRAM (transverse rectus abdominis) flap?
   A. Scar tissue that feels like recurrent cancer
   B. Abdominal wall hernia
   C. Persistent pain
   D. Capsular contracture
   E. Wound infection

## COMMENT

**Indications for mastectomy with breast reconstruction** • Often, a diagnosed breast cancer can be excised by lumpectomy and either axillary dissection or sentinel lymph node biopsy followed by chemotherapy or radiation therapy or both. In patients with small tumors, lumpectomy will give an aesthetically acceptable result, making it the procedure of choice in most patients. In this patient, a mastectomy followed by reconstruction is a much more aesthetically acceptable treatment because excision of a lump occupying 50% of the breast volume would leave an unacceptable result aesthetically. Neither the presence of cancer in the breast nor axillary dissection is a contraindication to reconstruction.

**Timing of chemotherapy, radiation therapy, and breast reconstruction** • Both chemotherapy and radiation therapy interfere with wound healing and should be delayed for at least 2 weeks after any major surgery. In practice, this is not an issue. After mastectomy the patient needs 2 weeks of postoperative recovery before either of these treatments can be started to allow the mastectomy incision to heal. Thus, breast reconstruction at the time of mastectomy does not unnecessarily delay adjunctive therapy for cancer. Once chemotherapy or radiation therapy is initiated, reconstruction should wait until at least 6 weeks after completion of treatment and until the white blood cell count has returned to normal. Although either delayed or immediate reconstruction is acceptable, immediate reconstruction is preferred for its improved aesthetic outcome.

**Complications of breast implant surgery** • Expander/implant reconstruction uses tissue expanders to expand the skin that is deficient after the mastectomy. Later, after adequate expansion, the expander is exchanged for a permanent implant, either silicone or saline filled. Benefits over TRAM flap include simplicity of surgery, patient comfort, and ability to choose breast size. Complications include up to a 20% clinically significant capsular contracture rate (approximately 5% require reoperation for this problem), infections (less than 5%), and extrusion of the implant (less than 2%). Excellent aesthetic results are achievable in small to medium breasts. Larger breast size may require a contralateral breast reduction, mastopexy, augmentation, or a combination of these to match symmetry. Bilateral mastectomy patients have excellent results after this type of reconstruction because it is easy to match symmetry.

**TRAM flap reconstruction** • Autologous tissue reconstruction options include a pedicled transverse rectus abdominis (TRAM) flap, a free TRAM flap, and a latissimus dorsi myocutaneous flap. Without an implant there is no risk of capsular contracture. TRAM flap reconstructions have their own problems, including ischemia of the flap, abdominal wall hernias, scar tissue formation that can clinically resemble a cancer recurrence, and chronic and persistent pain of the abdominal wall.

**Answers** • 1-E 2-E 3-A 4-D

## CASE PRESENTATION

A 68-year-old man with insulin-dependent diabetes presents to your office 2 weeks after sustaining a laceration to his right leg over the tibia when he tripped over a fallen tree limb in his yard. He has been treating the wound with hydrogen peroxide and dry dressings daily without success. He denies fever, chills, or excessive pain in the leg.

1. Which of the following are classic phases of wound healing?
   A. Inflammatory phase
   B. Repair phase
   C. Maturation phase
   D. Contraction phase
   E. A, B, and C
2. Which of the following can be described as the control cell of wound repair?
   A. Platelet
   B. Lymphocyte
   C. Polymorphonuclear leukocyte
   D. Macrophage
   E. Fibroblast
3. During wound healing, which type of cell produces collagen?
   A. Platelet
   B. Lymphocyte
   C. Polymorphonuclear leukocyte
   D. Macrophage
   E. Fibroblast
4. Of the following, which is the best method of cleaning the open wound on a daily basis?
   A. Hydrogen peroxide
   B. Soap and tap water
   C. Betadine solution
   D. Dakin's solution
   E. Acetic acid solution
5. The patient's wound fails to heal despite appropriate care. Bone is exposed at the base of the wound. Which of the following is the most appropriate method to achieve coverage of this patient's wound?
   A. Local myocutaneous flap
   B. Free myocutaneous flap
   C. Full-thickness skin graft
   D. Split-thickness skin graft
   E. Pig skin coverage followed by full-thickness skin graft

## COMMENT

**Phases of wound healing** • The classic phases of wound healing are (1) inflammatory, (2) repair, and (3) maturation. The inflammatory phase begins with a 5- to 10-minute transient period of vasoconstriction. Following this, platelets stick to exposed subendothelial collagen and then aggregate with other "activated" platelets. Platelet degranulation occurs, releasing platelet-derived growth factor (PDGF), adenosine diphosphate (ADP), transforming growth factor β (TGFβ), serotonins, fibronectins, and other growth factors. Vasodilation then occurs with the release of vasoactive substances, including eicosanoids, the key factor in the inflammatory phase. Loose adhesion of monocytes and polymorphonuclear leukocytes is mediated by selectins. Tighter adhesion leading to diapedesis is mediated by integrins. The repair phase (also known as the proliferative or fibroplasia phase) consists of angiogenesis, migration, secretion of ground substance, and collagen synthesis. This phase includes wound contracture and continues until the wound has closed and epithelialized. The maturation phase begins as early as 2 weeks following wounding. During this time, collagen fibers rearrange to improve the functional result.

**Control of wound healing** • The macrophage is the control cell of wound repair. Macrophages control growth factor production, cytokines, matrix production and degradation, angiogenesis, and epithelialization. Hypoxia, cytokines, and other peptides activate macrophages. Lymphocytes are not needed in wound healing.

**Collagen synthesis in wound healing** • During the repair phase there is migration of cells into the wound. Fibroblasts secrete first glycosaminoglycans and then collagen. Collagen is initially laid down in a random pattern. During the maturation phase, resorption of this collagen occurs and new collagen is laid down aligned along mechanical stress lines. Collagen content plateaus at about 6 weeks.

**Wound cleansing** • Regular mild, unscented soap along with tap water or irrigation with sterile saline are good methods of cleaning an open wound. Scrubbing should be avoided. Hydrogen peroxide and other antibacterial agents are cytotoxic and can impede wound healing when used on a chronic basis. As long as the wound is open and well vascularized, there is no need to enforce sterile conditions during wound care, although cross contamination between patients should be avoided.

**Wound coverage** • Skin grafts survive the first several days by obtaining nutrition and oxygen from serous fluid in the wound by a process called *imbibition*. Full-thickness grafts are aesthetically more attractive and contract much less than split-thickness grafts. Split-thickness grafts require less donor site area since they can be meshed and expanded. They can be contoured more easily, and the holes created when the graft is meshed allow drainage better than full-thickness grafts, which usually are not meshed. Physical separation of the graft by seroma or hematoma is the most common cause of skin graft loss. Because the split-thickness graft is better at drainage, and because it has less tissue mass to support during healing, it has a higher survival rate than the full-thickness graft. Exposed bone requires coverage with soft tissue to survive. If not covered, the bone will die from either infection (osteomyelitis) or from lack of blood supply. Skin grafts are inadequate to cover exposed bone. Both local and free muscle flaps are good coverage for bones. A local flap should be used if one is available because a free flap is a long and challenging procedure for both the patient and the surgeon.

**Answers** • 1-E 2-D 3-E 4-B 5-A

## CASE PRESENTATION

A 58-year-old retired lawyer presents with complaints of buttock and thigh "tiredness". His discomfort comes on after walking 100 yards, and he frequently sits or leans to get symptom relief. He denies impotence and has no other significant illnesses. He has no symptoms of coronary artery disease, though he has smoked one pack of cigarettes per day for 35 years.

1. Important risk factors for peripheral vascular disease would include:
   A. Diabetes mellitus, elevated cholesterol, and hypertension
   B. A grandfather with heart attack at age 68
   C. Elevated homocysteine levels
   D. All of the above
   E. A and C
2. Which of the following findings would be *most inconsistent* with a diagnosis of peripheral vascular disease?
   A. Normal palpable pulses
   B. Bilateral femoral bruits
   C. Normal ankle-brachial index (ABI)
   D. Palpable pulses and normal ankle-brachial index following heel raises for 2 minutes
   E. Negative straight leg raising test and normal ankle reflexes
3. Following your history and physical exam, you suspect vascular disease contributing to his symptoms. You would do the following:
   A. Obtain formal vascular laboratory segmental pressures and Doppler derived waveforms
   B. Request a duplex ultrasound of the abdominal aorta and iliacs
   C. Promptly obtain an arteriogram
   D. Recommend cessation of smoking and avoidance of exercise
   E. Consider pharmacologic treatment with pentoxifylline or cilostazol
4. The patient does not follow your recommendations and presents 6 months later with severely limiting cramping symptoms in his calves when walking. He also has pain in his toes and forefeet at night improved with dependency. His femoral pulses are markedly reduced and bilateral bruits are present. He has dependent rubor but no tissue breakdown or lesions. Which of the following are true?
   A. Without intervention, he is at high risk for limb loss, and an angiogram will be needed.
   B. His ABI will be about 0.6, and femoropopliteal bypassing will be needed.
   C. His symptoms may respond to angioplasty alone.
   D. All of the above.
   E. A and C.

## COMMENT

**Risk factors for atherosclerotic peripheral vascular disease (ASPVD)** • Accepted risk factors include diabetes mellitus, hypertension, lipid disorders, and a family history of early atherosclerosis (first-degree relatives, under 60 years old). Tobacco abuse, especially smoking, is the single most common risk factor encountered, especially in ASPVD before the age of 55. Obesity and alcohol use are not considered independent risk factors for ASPVD. Elevated homocysteine levels have been considered a risk factor for premature ASPVD whose effects can be ameliorated by folic acid and/or vitamin $B_6$ supplementation.

**Physical findings** • While diminished pulses or bruits in the lower extremities are clearly suspicious for peripheral vascular disease, ASPVD can also present with normal pulses and a normal ankle-brachial index (ABI) at rest. However, if pulses are palpable and the ABI is normal (equal or slightly greater than 1) after a few minutes of calf muscle exercise, this excludes a vascular etiology for symptoms. To evaluate possible neurologic causes for pain, a straight leg test should be performed and reflexes tested. Positive neurologic findings should decrease suspicion of a vascular etiology.

**Evaluation and management** • The natural history of claudication is generally benign, with limb loss in only about 5% of patients over 5 years. Angiography is indicated only when interventions, such as angioplasty or surgery, are entertained. These are usually considered only for the approximately 20% of patients with progressive, debilitating symptoms that limit the patient's quality of life, or when limb-threatening ischemia develops. In fact, patients with leg claudication due to ASPVD are much more likely to die from coronary artery disease than they are to lose a limb during the same period. Many patients with claudication will significantly improve if their risk factors, including smoking, are controlled and a regular progressive exercise program can be maintained. Pharmacologic treatment with either pentoxifylline or cilostazol has been successful in ameliorating symptoms in many patients, but is expensive, has side effects, and is not effective for all patients. These agents can be reserved for patients in whom other nonoperative management strategies fail. Duplex ultrasound of the aorta and iliac vessels has no role in initial evaluation and management of claudication, especially in a patient such as this whose symptoms suggest disease distal to these vessels. Formal segmental pressures and Doppler derived waveforms can provide important information confirming the location of ASPVD and a baseline measurement for prognosis and symptom progression.

**Limb-threatening ischemia** • Our patient developed symptoms and signs consistent with limb-threatening ischemia. Intervention is likely to be required to prevent tissue necrosis and gangrene with limb loss. ABI would be expected to be less than 0.4, although it may be less reliable in diabetic patients with falsely elevated values even in the setting of advanced ischemia. With reduced femoral pulses and femoral bruits, the likelihood of finding iliac disease amenable to angioplasty or stenting is greater. (Note that our patient has signs of femoral disease, so surgery would require aortofemoral bypass.) Femoropopliteal disease may be present, but angiography is usually needed to assess this component. Stent placement for this is not as effective as iliac angioplasty or bypass. If multilevel disease is contributory, symptoms can often be relieved with intervention at only the proximal level of obstruction and more distal intervention may not be required, as long as tissue necrosis is not present. Angiographic findings and physiologic function are more important in determining suitability for intervention than age, diabetes, or renal function.

**Answers** • 1-E 2-D 3-A 4-E

## CASE PRESENTATION

A 58-year-old retired lawyer is noted to have dilatation of the abdominal aorta found on CT scanning during evaluation for chronic low back pain.

1. Diagnosis of an abdominal aortic aneurysm (AAA) requires:
   A. Aorta diameter greater than 8 cm
   B. Aorta diameter more than 0.5 cm larger than the suprarenal aorta
   C. Aorta diameter more than 50% larger than the suprarenal aorta
   D. An aorta diameter increased more than 50% over the expected diameter
   E. Aorta diameter greater than 6 cm
2. Of the following, which is a recognized risk factor for development of AAA?
   A. Family history
   B. Hypertension
   C. Smoking
   D. Elevated cholesterol
   E. A, B, and C
3. When assessing an older patient for possible AAA, which of the following may be considered?
   A. The prevalence of AAA in men aged 65 to 75 is 10%.
   B. A family history of polycystic kidney disease increases the risk of AAA.
   C. Those with chronic obstructive pulmonary disease (COPD) and $\alpha_1$-antitrypsin deficiency have a higher risk of AAA.
   D. All of the above.
   E. A and C.
4. Which of the following is true regarding the etiology of AAA?
   A. Elastin and collagen are decreased in the walls of AAA compared with aortas with atherosclerotic occlusive disease.
   B. Atherosclerosis is the most common cause.
   C. Matrix metalloproteases are thought to be important in AAA development, and a tapering diameter from distal thoracic aorta to abdominal aorta and other mechanical factors seem to play a role.
   D. A and C.
   E. All of the above.
5. Physical examination and CT scan reveal a nontender 4.0-cm infrarenal AAA. Which of the following courses of action do you suggest?
   A. Elective Dacron graft repair via a transabdominal incision
   B. Serial ultrasound examinations in 3 to 6 months
   C. Stent graft repair via bilateral femoral cutdowns
   D. Serial CT scans every 3 to 6 months
   E. Propranolol and minocycline administration

## COMMENT

**Definition** • The accepted operational definition of an abdominal aortic aneurysm is an enlargement of the outside diameter of the artery more than 0.5 cm compared with the suprarenal aorta, or an aortic diameter greater than 4 cm. AAA is 3 to 4 times more prevalent among men than women, with a prevalence in men aged 65 to 74 of about 2%. Among patients with first-degree male relatives with AAA, the prevalence is over 10 times greater.

**Risk factors for AAA development** • The most important risk factors for AAA development, which are frequently present in these patients, are a history of smoking, family history of AAA, and hypertension. High cholesterol is not considered a major risk factor for this disease.

**Etiology of AAA** • The cause of AAA is not definitively established. However, it is probably not the same process that results in generalized atherosclerosis, although atherosclerosis is frequently associated. Recent evidence suggests that forms of serine proteases called matrix metalloproteases are involved; these effect the breakdown of elastin and collagen in the wall of the aorta. Mechanical factors—such as the tapering of the aorta—also may play a role. $\alpha_1$-Antitrypsin deficiency among patients with AAA and COPD has also been noted (a gee-whiz fact that has appeared on the boards).

**Management of small AAA** • The risk of aneurysm rupture increases exponentially with increasing aortic diameter. Aneurysms 4 cm or less in diameter have a relatively low annual risk of rupture of about 2%. This is approximately the mortality rate for elective repair. Therefore, the best option for a 4-cm AAA is usually serial observation with ultrasound, which is almost as accurate as CT, is much cheaper, and does not require contrast injection. While beta blockade and minocycline have been proposed as agents to reduce the rate of AAA enlargement, they have yet to be analyzed in prospective randomized trials. (Beta blockade does slow progression of thoracic aortic expansion and lower the risk of rupture in Marfan's syndrome.) Operative intervention is generally not warranted for asymptomatic AAA less than 5 cm in diameter. Above that, the risk of rupture is significant.

**Answers** • 1-B 2-E 3-C 4-D 5-B

## CASE PRESENTATION

A 62-year-old male patient being followed for a small (4.0 cm) asymptomatic abdominal aortic aneurysm (AAA) is found, 12 months later, to now have an aneurysm measuring 5.0 cm in transverse diameter on ultrasound.

1. His estimated risk of AAA rupture over the next 5 years is approximately:
   A. 10%
   B. 25%
   C. 50%
   D. 75%
   E. 95%
2. In patients undergoing elective repair of AAA, which of the following is true?
   A. Coronary artery disease is present in 35% to 50% of patients with AAA.
   B. Endovascular stent repair has a lower mortality and complication rate than standard open repair.
   C. Mortality of ruptured AAA repair is 50% to 75%, whereas elective repair is safe, with a 30-day mortality of 3% to 5%.
   D. All of the above are true.
   E. A and C are true.
3. On evaluation, you find that the aneurysm is quite tender. The patient complains of mid-back pain. Based on your exam and his complaints you feel this aneurysm is symptomatic. His risk of rupture is:
   A. 25% over the next 5 years
   B. 30% over the next month
   C. 30% over the next 6 months
   D. 50% over the next year
   E. Approximately the same as an asymptomatic aneurysm
4. Your next diagnostic test is:
   A. CT scan of the abdomen and pelvis
   B. Cardiac stress thallium evaluation
   C. Matrix metalloproteinase-9 level
   D. Abdominal ultrasound
   E. Aortography

## COMMENT

**Risk of rupture in larger aneurysms** • The risk of rupture of a 5-cm AAA over a 5-year period is about 5% per year. A good rule of thumb to determine the 5-year risk of rupture is to square the maximum diameter ( i.e., a 5-cm AAA has about a 25% 5-year risk, a 6-cm AAA a 36% 5-year risk, and so on). Since the mean annual growth rate of an AAA is 3 to 5 mm per year, a rate of enlargement faster than this may increase the risk of rupture as well.

**Risk of AAA repair** • Coronary artery disease is prevalent among patients with AAA, present in 35% to 50%, even in the absence of symptoms. The mortality of ruptured AAA is extremely high (50% to 70%) even if the patients make it to the hospital alive, hence the rationale for elective repair, which has a relatively low mortality when performed by experienced vascular surgeons. Interestingly, endovascular repair using stent graft devices deployed via operative cutdown on the femoral artery has not yet demonstrated a convincing reduction in mortality and morbidity compared with standard open repair, and the durability of stenting is uncertain. We may expect this new technique to evolve.

**Symptomatic AAA** • An aneurysm accompanied by abdominal or back pain, or an aneurysm that is tender on examination, carries a high risk of imminent rupture. Nearly one-third of these "symptomatic aneurysms" rupture within 1 month, and nearly two-thirds rupture within 6 months. Most symptomatic aneurysms will rupture within a year. The maximum diameter is not a primary determinate of rupture for symptomatic AAA.

**Evaluation of symptomatic AAA** • The best available diagnostic test for a symptomatic AAA is a CT scan, preferably with intravenous contrast, to assess the extent of the aneurysm and to detect any evidence of rupture.

**Answers** • 1-B 2-E 3-B 4-A

## CASE PRESENTATION

A 35-year-old female architect develops sudden onset of painful left calf swelling the morning after a 4-hour-long airline flight. She has no previous history of leg swelling, although her mother did. She has no children and is on oral contraceptives. She does not smoke or have any other known illnesses. On physical exam she has a tender, swollen calf with 3+ pitting edema. Homans' sign is negative.

1. The most useful method to diagnose deep venous thrombosis (DVT) is:
   A. Clinical examination
   B. Venogram
   C. Duplex Doppler ultrasound
   D. Magnetic resonance angiography (MRA)
   E. None of the above
2. Which of the following statements regarding deep venous thrombosis is true?
   A. In patients with lower extremity varicosities, "stripping" of the saphenous vein can reduce the risk of deep vein thrombosis.
   B. Contrast venography is required before initiating therapy for DVT.
   C. Factors thought to be necessary for development of DVT include intimal injury to the vein, stasis of blood in the vein, and hypercoagulability.
   D. DVT does not lead to later development of venous stasis ulcers.
   E. None of the above.
3. Which of the following would be an appropriate alternative to unfractionated heparin in the initial management of this patient?
   A. Low-molecular-weight heparin, dose-adjusted for weight
   B. Aspirin
   C. Catheter-directed thrombolysis
   D. Inferior vena cava filter placement
   E. Open thromboembolectomy
4. Aside from detection of DVT, other indications for duplex Doppler study include:
   A. Evaluation of cerebrovascular disease
   B. Initial evaluation of intermittent claudication
   C. Renal artery exam when renovascular hypertension is suspected
   D. All of the above
   E. A and C

## COMMENT

**Diagnosis of deep venous thrombosis** • The clinical diagnosis of deep venous thrombosis is unreliable, even among apparently symptomatic patients. Homans' sign (calf pain with passive dorsiflexion of the foot) is overrated as a diagnostic maneuver. The presence of thrombus in the deep venous system diminishes the venous flow detectable by both continuous wave Doppler and pulse wave duplex Doppler. Although continuous wave Doppler can be used at the bedside to heighten clinical suspicion, the most accurate and useful test to diagnose and localize DVT is duplex Doppler ultrasound, which will demonstrate a noncompressible vein with loss of flow variation and augmentation over the respiratory cycle and during maneuvers that empty the venous system. MRA is not a practical or cost-effective exam for diagnosis of DVT. Doppler evaluation has replaced contrast venography as the initial study.

**Management, sequelae, and pathophysiology of DVT** • DVT is thought to begin in vessels with intimal injury and stasis. Hypercoagulability is also thought to be important. DVT can damage the valves of the deep venous system, leading to later development of venous stasis ulcers and skin changes. Duplex ultrasound is accurate, and contrast venography is not needed before initiating therapy unless the duplex is equivocal. For many years, DVT therapy included continuous administration of intravenous (unfractionated) heparin to prolong the partial thromboplastin time to at least twice normal, followed by oral warfarin for at least 3, and preferably 6, months.

Varicose veins result from valvular incompetence of the *superficial* venous system. Pain or bleeding can result. Severe symptoms may be relieved by vein stripping. Superficial vein stripping has no influence on the factors that lead to development of DVT and has no role in the treatment or prevention of DVT.

**Treatment options** • Outpatient use of low-molecular-weight heparin given subcutaneously once or twice daily while oral anticoagulation is adjusted is effective. Antiplatelet agents, such as aspirin, are inadequate therapy for acute DVT. Surgical thrombectomy remains controversial because of the propensity for re-occlusion. Thrombolysis with various tissue plasminogen activators appears to be as efficacious as heparin in prevention of pulmonary embolus, but the high bleeding risk keeps it from being first-line therapy. Inferior vena cava filters are generally not indicated for DVT unless there is a contraindication to anticoagulation or a complication resulting from it. Failure of anticoagulation therapy (i.e., pulmonary embolus despite anticoagulation) may be another indication for filter placement.

**Duplex Doppler** • The greatest utility of duplex Doppler, which includes a B-mode ultrasound image and Doppler ultrasound that allows for focused sampling of flow velocities within a vessel, lies in the evaluation of cerebrovascular disease, the diagnosis of deep venous thrombosis, and follow-up of lower extremity autogenous vein bypasses. Evaluation of renal artery stenosis can also be accomplished with a high degree of precision in experienced vascular laboratories. Its role in the management of lower extremity arterial occlusive disease is not as clear. While it may play an adjunctive role in helping to decide when and where intervention is appropriate, it currently has no clear role in the initial management of patients presenting with lower extremity claudication symptoms.

**Answers** • 1-C 2-C 3-A 4-E

## CASE PRESENTATION

A 65-year-old former smoker is noted to have a left carotid bruit on physical examination during routine evaluation of his essential hypertension. He has no history of vision loss, lateralizing motor weakness, or sensory deficit, and no history of aphasia. His father had a stroke at age 67.

1. Which of the following would be indicated at this time?
   A. Arrange for computed tomography of the brain, with and without contrast
   B. Cerebral angiography and angioplasty/stenting
   C. Administration of clopidogrel (Plavix)
   D. Duplex ultrasound of the cerebral vessels
   E. Carotid endarterectomy
2. He is found to have an internal carotid stenosis of greater than 80% of its diameter. Which of the following is true?
   A. There is little risk of stroke if he is maintained on aspirin.
   B. In the absence of symptoms, he will not benefit from prophylactic carotid endarterectomy.
   C. There is no substitute for cerebral angiography prior to intervention.
   D. He has a high likelihood of having concomitant coronary artery disease.
   E. He must have an expected life span of at least 10 years to have a survival benefit from carotid endarterectomy.
3. The patient ignores your advice and returns after 12 months with two distinct recent episodes of transient ischemic attacks with right arm weakness and an expressive aphasia. Both attacks resolved within minutes. The Doppler study shows no change in his internal carotid artery. Which of the following is definitive therapy?
   A. Heparin anticoagulation followed by oral warfarin
   B. Initiate oral warfarin
   C. Carotid endarterectomy
   D. Add clopidogrel to his daily aspirin
   E. Carotid artery bypass surgery

## COMMENT

**Evaluation of asymptomatic carotid bruit** • There is no clinical benefit for computed tomography (CT) of the brain in an asymptomatic patient with a neck bruit. Cerebral angiography is not indicated in an asymptomatic patient, and certainly not without first confirming the presence of a significant stenosis. Duplex ultrasound is the best diagnostic screening test for determining the hemodynamic significance and stroke risk of an asymptomatic carotid bruit.

**Management of asymptomatic carotid stenosis** • Asymptomatic patients with significant carotid stenosis are at increased risk for stroke, despite medical management with aspirin. However, the stroke risk is still somewhat less than 20% over several years. Carotid endarterectomy clearly has a role in stroke prevention for otherwise good-risk patients who have a life expectancy of at least 2 years, when the stenosis is greater than or equal to 70% of the vessel's diameter. It reduces the stroke risk 3 to 5 times compared with medical therapy. With less severe stenosis, there is little benefit from surgical correction, and antiplatelet therapy is indicated. To date, carotid angioplasty and stent placement holds no clear benefit over carotid endarterectomy in terms of stroke reduction, hospitalization, or costs.

Prior to carotid endarterectomy, high-quality duplex scanning is increasingly used as a substitute for cerebral angiography among asymptomatic patients. Carotid endarterectomy should never be offered for carotid bruit alone. Concomitant coronary artery disease is common among patients with carotid disease. In fact, the risk of a myocardial infarction in this group is higher than the risk of stroke.

**Management of symptomatic carotid stenosis** • Patients with symptomatic transient ischemic attacks (TIAs) and carotid stenosis exceeding 70% clearly benefit from carotid endarterectomy. Endarterectomy has such a clear benefit over medical therapy in this setting that it should be offered to all but extremely debilitated patients. Neither heparin anticoagulation, increased aspirin dosage, or warfarin has been shown to be of benefit for intermittent TIAs, though warfarin or clopidogrel may be considered for patients who are not surgical candidates. Magnetic resonance imaging of the brain has limited utility in the patient who does not have a persistent neurologic deficit, although magnetic resonance angiography may complement duplex scanning and/or replace standard cerebral contrast angiography for evaluation of the carotid vessels.

**Answers** • 1-D 2-D 3-C

## CASE PRESENTATION

A 33-year-old woman develops acute right lower quadrant pain, nausea, and vomiting while at work. The pain is colicky in nature and radiates into the groin region. Other aspects of her history are unremarkable. On physical examination, she is noted to be afebrile and her vital signs are within normal limits. Her abdomen is not tender and there are no obvious masses present. Urine analysis reveals 2 to 4 white blood cells per high-power field and 8 to 10 red blood cells per high-power field.

1. The most logical next step in the evaluation of this patient would be:
   A. Contrasted CT scan of the abdomen and pelvis
   B. Serum (or urine) pregnancy test
   C. Intravenous pyelogram (IVP)
   D. Serum creatinine measurement
   E. Laparoscopy with appendectomy
2. Computed tomographic intravenous pyelogram (CTIVP) reveals a 3-mm stone in the distal right ureter. There is minimal hydronephrosis and a normal contralateral kidney. Pain is well controlled on narcotic pain medicine. The most logical next step would be:
   A. Extracorporeal shock-wave lithotripsy (ESWL)
   B. Ureteroscopic stone extraction
   C. Symptomatic treatment with urologic follow-up
   D. Admission to the hospital for pain management
   E. Open stone removal
3. The most common stone composition found in patients in the United States is:
   A. Calcium phosphate
   B. Calcium oxalate
   C. Magnesium ammonium phosphate
   D. Uric acid
   E. Mixed cholesterol
4. Which of the following would be the best course of action for this patient to avoid kidney stones in the future?
   A. Low-salt diet
   B. Low-calcium diet
   C. Low-fat diet
   D. Increased fluid intake
   E. No therapy will influence stone formation

## COMMENT

**Evaluation of the patient with ureteral stones** • Pregnancy must be ruled out before proceeding with diagnostic studies utilizing ionizing radiation. Although ultrasound does not expose patients to ionizing radiation, it is not as accurate as other modalities in diagnosing urolithiasis. Laparoscopy would be indicated only if an acute surgical condition, such as acute appendicitis, were suspected. This patient has no physical findings consistent with peritoneal irritation. Further evidence would be needed before presuming a diagnosis of appendicitis and proceeding with surgery. Of the imaging studies mentioned, IVP, after a negative pregnancy test, would be the study of choice. Serum creatinine measurement should be obtained to assess the patient's renal function before administering iodinated contrast material. *Contrasted* CT scans are not useful for the diagnosis of stone disease. *Noncontrasted* spiral CT scan (CTIVP), however, is as sensitive and specific for stone disease as a standard IVP without the risks of iodine contrast. This study has largely replaced IVP in diagnosis of urolithiasis in the emergency setting. Interpretation requires an experienced radiologist, however.

**Management of ureteral stones** • The best management for this patient would be symptomatic treatment alone. Stones up to 4 mm will pass spontaneously in approximately 90% of patients. Stone disease is extremely painful, and symptomatic therapy should take this into consideration. Extracorporeal shock-wave lithotripsy is difficult for distal ureteral stones due to overlying pelvic bones. Some studies also suggest that ovarian damage may occur in female patients. Ureteroscopic stone extraction requires anesthesia and would be indicated only in unusual circumstances, such as in a patient with a solitary kidney and progressive renal insufficiency, a patient with unremitting pain, or failure to pass the stone in a reasonable amount of time. Open stone surgery is rarely indicated. Admission is only indicated for unremitting pain or vomiting, fevers, or accompanying renal insufficiency. Any patient with stone disease and fevers constitutes a urologic emergency and requires immediate evaluation by a urologist.

**Stone types** • Calcium oxalate stones make up 33% of the stones in the United States and are the most common single stone type. Mixed calcium oxalate and calcium phosphate stones are also frequently found. Magnesium ammonium phosphate (struvite) stones, which are associated with urea splitting organisms and infection, constitute 15% of stones. Uric acid stones and cystine stones constitute approximately 8% and 3% of stones, respectively. Cystine stones are associated with cystinuria, a genetic recessive trait. Mixed cholesterol stones occur in the biliary tree, not in the urinary tract.

**Stone prevention** • Increased fluid intake, in the form of water, is the only therapy proven to decrease stone formation. Because stone formation is dependent on salt precipitation, the resultant increased urine production will decrease the incidence of stone formation. Decreased calcium intake has been advocated in the past. However, this has now been proven to be counterproductive. Calcium binds oxalate in the small intestine, and decreased calcium may actually increase oxalate uptake from the bowel and thus increase urinary oxalate. Low-fat diets have no proven effect on stone formation.

**Answers** • 1-B 2-C 3-B 4-D

## CASE PRESENTATION

A 32-year-old woman presents with a palpable 2-cm, nontender mass in the left lobe of her thyroid.

1. Which of the following statements about thyroid nodules is true?
   A. Thyroid nodules are more common in men than in women.
   B. Thyroid nodules are commonly reported in autopsies in patients with no history of thyroid disease.
   C. Approximately 30% of solitary thyroid nodules are malignant.
   D. Most thyroid nodules are functional.
   E. The most common type of thyroid nodule is papillary carcinoma.
2. Which of the following would suggest a benign nodule?
   A. Unilateral cervical lymphadenopathy
   B. Hoarseness
   C. History of previous neck irradiation
   D. Episodic headaches and hypertension
   E. Palpitations, heat intolerance, and weight loss
3. Of the following, which is needed to determine the type of nodule?
   A. Fine needle aspiration biopsy
   B. Ultrasound of the mass
   C. Nuclear scan of the thyroid
   D. Magnetic resonance imaging (MRI) study of the neck
   E. Computed tomography (CT) of the neck
4. Which of the following is the most common complication of unilateral thyroid lobectomy?
   A. Hoarseness
   B. Hypocalcemia
   C. Trousseau's sign
   D. Seizures
   E. Chvostek's sign

## COMMENT

**Thyroid nodules** • Thyroid nodules are more common in women than in men and are, in fact, very common. Autopsy series reveal that up to 50% of people have thyroid nodules. Typically, only those that are palpable need to be evaluated. Even when palpable, solitary nodules are benign approximately 95% of the time, and most are not functional. The most common type of nodule is a colloid nodule.

**Characteristics of malignant nodules** • Functional nodules are rarely malignant. Hoarseness suggests malignant invasion of the recurrent laryngeal nerve. A history of radiation exposure is a recognized predisposing factor for thyroid malignancy. Ipsilateral lymphadenopathy suggests metastatic spread. Episodic hypertension and headaches are symptoms of pheochromocytoma. While rare, multiple endocrine neoplasia type II (MEN II) must be considered. MEN type IIA consists of medullary thyroid carcinoma, pheochromocytoma, and parathyroid hyperplasia. MEN type IIB includes medullary thyroid carcinoma, pheochromocytoma, and mucosal neuromas.

**Diagnosis of thyroid mass** • Fine needle aspiration biopsy is the initial best choice. Ultrasound can distinguish solid from cystic masses, but benign and malignant masses can be cystic. Thyroid nuclear scan can be used to assess the functional activity of a thyroid mass but cannot determine if the mass is malignant. CT and MRI of the neck will not distinguish benign from malignant masses until the malignancy is advanced and has invaded surrounding structures.

**Complications of thyroid surgery** • Damage to the recurrent laryngeal nerve and the parathyroid glands may occur with thyroidectomy. Hypoparathyroidism leads to hypocalcemia, which, in turn, causes a form of tetany (positive Trousseau's and Chvostek's signs). However, with resection of only one thyroid lobe, hypocalcemia would not be expected because the contralateral parathyroid glands are adequate to maintain calcium homeostasis. Unilateral recurrent laryngeal nerve injury can occur during unilateral thyroid lobectomy, causing hoarseness.

**Answers** • 1-B 2-E 3-A 4-A

## CASE PRESENTATION

A 60-year-old man with a single nodule on the left lobe of his thyroid gland undergoes needle aspiration biopsy.

1. If cytology on the resulting specimen revealed a cellular aspirate with predominantly follicular cells, which of the following would be the most appropriate next step in management?
   A. Left thyroid lobectomy
   B. Total thyroidectomy
   C. Radiation therapy followed by total thyroidectomy
   D. Thyroid hormone suppression therapy
   E. Radioactive iodine ($^{131}$I) therapy
2. In this case, a unilateral thyroid lobectomy is performed, and the lesion proves to be malignant. A chest x-ray reveals several nodules in the lungs consistent with metastatic disease. What is the next step in management?
   A. Cervical lymph node dissection and completion thyroidectomy
   B. Completion thyroidectomy alone
   C. Radioactive iodine therapy
   D. Completion thyroidectomy, radioactive iodine ablation therapy, and thyroid hormone suppression therapy
   E. Completion thyroidectomy, cervical lymph node dissection, radioactive iodine therapy, and thyroid hormone suppression therapy
3. Which of the following would be most associated with a poor prognosis in a patient with papillary thyroid cancer?
   A. Cervical lymph node metastases
   B. Male patient 35 years of age
   C. Female patient 46 years of age
   D. A lesion with extension beyond the thyroid capsule
   E. A lesion 2.5 cm in diameter
4. Appropriate follow-up includes:
   A. Serial ultrasound examinations of the neck
   B. Annual computed tomographic scan of the neck
   C. Serial thyroglobulin levels in conjunction with radionuclide thyroid scans
   D. Annual radionuclide thyroid scan
   E. Serial thyroid function tests

## COMMENT

**Follicular thyroid cancer** • In patients with a follicular neoplasm, fine needle aspiration biopsy and cytology cannot distinguish follicular adenoma from follicular carcinoma. The presence of follicular cells in a thyroid mass mandates more definitive measures to assess for malignancy. A thyroid lobectomy would be indicated. The other measures listed would not be appropriate in the absence of a definitive diagnosis of thyroid malignancy.

**Management of follicular thyroid cancer** • Once diagnosed with malignancy, completion thyroidectomy is indicated because foci of malignancy in the other lobe are common. Radioactive iodine therapy is indicated for treatment of metastatic papillary and follicular thyroid cancers because these malignancies actively take up iodine. Completion thyroidectomy prevents the administered radioactive iodine from being bound in the remaining thyroid gland, making it available for uptake by any metastatic lesions. Cervical lymph node dissection is typically recommended only in the presence of palpable adenopathy. Both follicular thyroid cancers and papillary thyroid cancers also respond to suppression with thyroid hormone therapy and would be indicated in this patient. However, this should not be given concurrently with radioactive iodine because the exogenous thyroid hormone will suppress uptake of the radioactive iodine being administered for treatment. Anaplastic thyroid cancers and medullary thyroid cancers do not take up iodine, nor do they respond to thyroid hormone suppression.

**Prognostic factors in thyroid malignancy** • Poor prognostic factors in papillary thyroid malignancy include extension through the capsule of the gland, tumor size greater than 4 cm, age greater than 40 in men, and age greater than 50 in women. Unlike other malignancies, lymph node metastases do not alter prognosis in this condition.

**Follow-up of thyroid malignancy** • The goal of follow-up is identification of disease progression. Both follicular thyroid cancers and papillary thyroid cancers take up iodine. Therefore, thyroid scanning is a useful method to identify foci of recurrent and metastatic disease. However, prior to scanning, thyroid hormone suppression should be stopped to allow for uptake of the administered radioactive contrast agent. Another option occasionally used is to continue thyroid hormone replacement therapy but administer recombinant thyroid stimulating hormone (TSH) prior to scanning to allow uptake of the tracer despite the presence of thyroid hormone. Thyroglobulin levels may also serve as valuable tumor markers in these lesions. After a total thyroidectomy, thyroglobulin levels should be very low. An increase in thyroglobulin levels is suggestive of tumor recurrence and would justify thyroid scanning to localize any new or recurrent lesions.

**Answers** • 1-A 2-D 3-D 4-C

## CASE PRESENTATION

A 33-year-old woman presents with a palpable left breast mass she discovered while showering.

1. Which of the following would be most consistent with a benign lesion?
   A. Early age at menarche
   B. Maternal first cousin with breast cancer
   C. Nipple retraction
   D. Eczema-like changes on the areola
   E. Changes in the size of the mass with stage of the menstrual cycle
2. The patient reports a family history of breast cancer but no other history suggestive of malignancy. Physical examination reveals a 2.5-cm mass deep in the upper outer breast quadrant. Of the following, which is the most appropriate next step in management?
   A. Axillary lymph node sampling
   B. Needle localization breast biopsy
   C. Incisional biopsy of the mass
   D. Complete excision of the mass
   E. Modified radical mastectomy
3. A fibroadenoma is diagnosed. Further management should include:
   A. Yearly mammograms
   B. Axillary lymph node sampling
   C. Radical mastectomy
   D. Reassurance with instruction in breast self-examination and routine mammography
   E. Mirror-image biopsy of the opposite breast
4. Which of the following statements about mammography is true?
   A. Mammography should always be performed before excision of a palpable breast mass.
   B. Initial screening mammograms should be performed at age 30.
   C. Annual mammograms are recommended for women beginning at 45 to 50 years of age.
   D. Mammographic findings of a large single calcification are suggestive of carcinoma in situ.
   E. Mammography of the opposite breast should be performed in any patient diagnosed with carcinoma in situ in the opposite breast.

## COMMENT

**Characteristics of benign and malignant lesions** • Of the choices listed, only variation in the size of the mass over the patient's menstrual cycle is consistent with benign lesions. Family history is an important risk factor for malignancy. Although history of breast malignancy in a first-degree relative would be more significant, the presence of breast malignancy in any blood relative increases risk. Early age at menarche is also associated with an increased risk of breast malignancy. Nipple retraction is sometimes present in malignancy because fibrosis within the tumor causes contraction of the supporting structures. Paget's disease of the breast is a malignant condition characterized by changes on the nipple and areola that resemble eczema. A mass may or may not be palpable beneath the nipple. Eczematous changes on the nipple or areola always warrant evaluation for malignancy.

**Management of a palpable breast mass** • Palpable masses are best managed with excisional biopsy, not incisional biopsy. Needle localization is necessary only for nonpalpable lesions identified on mammography. Lymph node sampling and mastectomy are not necessary until malignancy is confirmed.

**Fibroadenoma** • Fibroadenoma is a benign condition requiring no further therapy. In the past, it was recommended that patients with fibrocystic disease avoid caffeine intake. However, there is minimal evidence to support this. Patients with a history of fibroadenoma are prone to development of new fibroadenomas. Reassurance and instruction in self-examination to identify future lesions as well as routine mammography are all that is required.

**Mammography** • Mammography is performed to identify malignancies in an early stage before they are palpable. Once a palpable mass is identified, mammography adds little to management of the mass, although it may be indicated to assess for other malignant foci. Small clusters of tiny calcifications are suggestive of malignancy, rather than single large calcifications. Current recommendations are for an initial baseline screening mammogram at 40 to 45 years of age and yearly screening mammograms beginning at age 45 to 50, depending on the patient's family history of breast cancer.

**Answers** • 1-E 2-D 3-D 4-C

## CASE PRESENTATION

A 62-year-old woman with no family history of breast disease presents with a 2.2-cm slightly painful mass in the upper outer quadrant of her left breast.

1. Of the following, which is the most appropriate next step in this patient's management?
   A. A trial of nonsteroidal anti-inflammatory agents
   B. Needle localization breast biopsy
   A. Immediate modified radical mastectomy
   C. Lumpectomy
   D. Lumpectomy and axillary node dissection
2. Ultimately, the patient is diagnosed with infiltrating ductal carcinoma. Lymph nodes are positive for metastatic disease. Which of the following statements about estrogen receptors is true?
   A. The presence of estrogen receptors in the tumor is a poor prognostic indicator.
   B. Estrogen receptor–positive tumors can be managed without radiation therapy.
   C. Estrogen receptors are present in over 80% of breast malignancies.
   D. Patients with estrogen receptor–positive tumors benefit from tamoxifen regardless of their age.
   E. Estrogen receptor–positive lesions are more prone to local recurrence.
3. The patient is found to have three positive freely movable lymph nodes. There is no evidence of distant metastases. Which of these is the correct staging description?
   A. T1, N2, M0
   B. T2, N1, M0
   C. T2, N2, M0
   D. T1, N2, M1
   E. T2, N1, M1
4. Which of the following would be the most appropriate treatment in this patient?
   A. Radiation therapy to the remaining left breast tissue
   B. Modified radical mastectomy without subsequent chemotherapy
   C. Radiation therapy to the remaining breast tissue and axilla, chemotherapy, and tamoxifen therapy
   D. Chemotherapy alone
   E. Modified radical mastectomy, radiation therapy, chemotherapy, and tamoxifen therapy

## COMMENT

**Evaluation of breast masses** • Breast cancers usually present as a nonpainful mass. However, on occasion they may be somewhat tender, and any breast mass must be regarded as a potentially malignant lesion, especially in this age group. There is no role for anti-inflammatory agents in evaluation or treatment of a breast mass. Needle localization breast biopsy would not be necessary in this patient because the mass is palpable. Modified radical mastectomy is not indicated unless malignancy has been proven and, even then, not without presenting the patient with other options for treatment. Excision of the mass is essential. Axillary lymph node dissection carries a significant morbidity and, like mastectomy, should not be performed until malignancy is proven.

**Estrogen receptors** • The presence of estrogen and progesterone receptors on a malignant breast mass is an indicator of a better prognosis and suggests that the cells in the malignant lesion are still fairly well differentiated and able to bind hormones that normally stimulate growth of breast tissue. Blocking of these receptors with tamoxifen will eliminate this ongoing hormonal stimulation of growth and assist in slowing tumor progression. In the past, it was felt that estrogen receptor–positive tumors in postmenopausal women would not benefit from anti-estrogen therapy. This is no longer felt to be true. Unfortunately, estrogen receptors are present in only 50% to 60% of tumors. The presence of these receptors does not alter the need for chemotherapy for treatment of distant disease or radiation for control of local disease. There is no evidence to suggest that local recurrence is more common in estrogen receptor–positive tumors.

**Breast cancer staging** • The TNM system has become the standard for staging of breast cancer and other tumors. T1 lesions are invasive lesions less than 2 cm in diameter. T2 lesions are 2 to 5 cm in diameter, while T3 lesions are greater than 5 cm in diameter. T4 tumors are those that invade the skin or invade into the chest wall. The presence of cancer cells in freely movable axillary lymph nodes would make this lesion an N1 lesion. In an N2 lesion, lymph nodes are fixed or matted within the axilla. In N3 lesions, the ipsilateral internal mammary nodes are involved. This patient has no distant metastases, making this an M0 lesion. Patients with distant metastases are considered to have an M1 lesion. (The application of this staging system with multiple solid tumors makes it a more likely board question—Case 14 involving colon cancer asks a similar question.)

**Adjuvant therapy in breast cancer** • The presence of tumor in the patient's lymph nodes suggests distant spread, which will require the use of chemotherapeutic agents. Because her tumor is estrogen receptor–positive, anti-estrogen therapy is also indicated. It is also important to assure local disease control. Either radiation therapy to the involved breast after lumpectomy with an adequate margin should be performed, or the patient should undergo modified radical mastectomy. Both are not required, although preoperative chemotherapy may be used to reduce tumor size and allow resection with adequate margins. This is especially true for patients with inflammatory breast cancer. The choice to pursue segmental resection with postoperative radiation versus modified radical resection needs to be discussed with the patient because some women will prefer mastectomy to avoid having to undergo radiation treatments.

**Answers** • 1-D 2-D 3-B 4-C

## CASE PRESENTATION

On a routine mammogram, a 52-year-old woman is found to have an area of stippled calcification in the upper outer quadrant of the right breast. No masses are palpable on examination.

1. Which of the following would be the most appropriate next step?
   A. Core biopsy with needle localization biopsy and sentinel lymph node biopsy if the core biopsy is positive for invasive malignancy
   B. Total mastectomy
   C. Excision of the upper outer quadrant of the right breast
   D. Reexamination in 3 months
   E. Needle localization breast biopsy with axillary lymph node dissection
2. The patient ultimately undergoes biopsy and is diagnosed with ductal carcinoma in situ (DCIS). The lesion is 1 cm in diameter and extends to within 1 mm of the biopsy specimen margin. Which of the following would be the most appropriate next step in management?
   A. Reexcision of the original biopsy site
   B. Reexcision of the original site with axillary lymph node dissection
   C. Reexcision of the biopsy site and sentinel lymph node biopsy
   D. Sentinel lymph node biopsy alone
   E. Reassurance and careful mammographic and physical examination follow-up
3. No evidence of invasive disease is identified. What would be the most appropriate next step in management?
   A. Total mastectomy
   B. Mirror-image biopsy of the opposite breast
   C. Bilateral total mastectomy
   D. Radiation therapy to the involved breast
   E. Follow-up with a repeat mammogram in 6 months and careful breast self-examination

## COMMENT

**Evaluation of mammographic abnormalities** • Stippled calcifications on mammography are considered suggestive of malignancy and require evaluation. A tissue diagnosis is essential to plan further therapy. However, definitive and staging procedures such as mastectomy and lymph node dissection should not be performed until malignancy has been confirmed with a tissue specimen. In this situation, needle localization breast biopsy will be required because the lesion is not palpable. However, core biopsy performed prior to needle localization may help with planning. If the core biopsy reveals invasive carcinoma, needle localization for excision of the lesion and sentinel lymph node biopsy can be performed simultaneously, avoiding the need for multiple surgical procedures. If the core biopsy shows no malignancy or shows evidence of in situ malignancy, no lymph node biopsy would be needed unless the final specimen demonstrates invasive cancer not seen on the core biopsy.

**Ductal carcinoma in situ** • DCIS is considered a precursor of invasive cancer but, because it has not penetrated through the basement membrane, metastatic spread will not have occurred. Therefore, there is no need to evaluate the axillary lymph nodes for evidence of metastatic spread. However, an adequate margin of normal breast beyond the lesion should be included in the excision. While most would agree that 1 cm is an adequate margin, some surgeons are beginning to accept less. Few, however, would accept a margin of only 1 mm. Therefore, in this situation, reexcision of the area would be appropriate to ensure an adequate tumor-free margin.

**Follow-up for DCIS** • Because excision of DCIS is considered curative, no further therapy is required. In the past, mirror-image biopsy of the opposite breast was recommended, particularly for patients with lobular carcinoma in situ. However, because screening methods have improved, this is no longer considered necessary. Patients with DCIS are at increased risk for development of breast cancer in the future, as are patients with lobular carcinoma in situ. Routine mammography and breast self-examination are essential to ensure early detection of malignancy in these relatively high-risk patients.

**Answers** • 1-A 2-A 3-E

## CASE PRESENTATION

A child born 6 weeks prematurely is now almost ready to go home. In preparing to discharge the child, the pediatrician notices that the child has a large right inguinal hernia. It is easily reducible and there has been no evidence of incarceration.

1. The parents are very anxious to take their baby home. The doctor should:
   A. Discharge the child with follow-up in the surgeon's office when the child reaches 50 weeks' gestation age
   B. Ask the surgeon to see the patient so that outpatient repair can be arranged in several weeks
   C. Discharge the child with follow-up with the surgeon in 6 months to see if the hernia has closed spontaneously
   D. Ask the surgeon to see the patient now so that repair can be arranged prior to discharge
   E. Order an ultrasound before discharge to make sure that there is no chance of incarceration
2. Nothing is done and, 6 months later, the infant presents with a 5-hour history of irritability, abdominal tenderness, fever, and a bulge in the right inguinal region. The clinical finding most consistent with incarcerated inguinal hernia is:
   A. Enlarged soft tissue fullness of the right hemiscrotum
   B. Irreducible bulge just above and lateral to the level of the base of the penis
   C. Tenderness focused on the ipsilateral testis, which rides higher than the contralateral testis
   D. Fluid-filled sac filling the right inguinal canal which transilluminates
   E. Persistent vomiting with right-sided abdominal tenderness
3. If this were a female infant with an asymptomatic, incarcerated, nontender, discrete mass in an inguinal hernia sac, which of the following would be the most likely identity of the mass?
   A. Bladder
   B. Fallopian tube
   C. Ovary
   D. Omentum
   E. Small intestine

## COMMENT

**Hernia in premature infants** • Inguinal hernias in premature infants have a relatively high risk of incarceration. The safest plan is to arrange for repair prior to discharge by a surgeon comfortable performing repair of hernias in very small infants. Inguinal hernias do not close spontaneously, as would be expected for an umbilical hernia in a child younger than 5 years of age. Diagnosis of an inguinal hernia is made clinically; ultrasound does not offer any additional information in this setting, nor can it be used to predict the risk of incarceration. In many cases, elective outpatient surgery on infants is postponed until after the child has reached 50 weeks' gestational age to reduce the risk of postoperative apnea. In this situation, however, the most prudent plan to avoid both the risk of incarceration and of apnea would be to arrange for surgery at least 24 hours prior to discharge. The parents are usually understanding.

**Incarcerated inguinal hernia** • Fullness in the scrotum or around the testis is not specific for incarcerated inguinal hernia in the absence of a bulge at the internal inguinal ring. The symptoms of fever, irritability, and a tender bulge at the internal ring strongly suggest incarcerated inguinal hernia. Prompt reduction of the contents of a recently incarcerated hernia back into the peritoneal cavity is necessary to avoid ischemia of the hernia contents, most likely bowel. Isolated tenderness of the testis alone (C), often accompanied by erythema, fever, and a high-riding testis, suggests a diagnosis of testicular torsion. Both symptomatic incarcerated inguinal hernia and testicular torsion warrant immediate surgical or urologic consultation. Irreversible ischemia may result from delay. A hydrocele may present as a cystic collection of fluid that may surround the testicle or fill the inguinal canal. Transillumination of a firm cystic mass is a simple test that may confirm the diagnosis of a hydrocele and differentiate the mass from a solid structure. Needle aspiration of a hydrocele, however, is not appropriate for diagnosis, because the fluid of a hydrocele usually recurs, and needle aspirate of a loop of bowel or solid tumor mass would result in contamination.

**Inguinal hernia in the female infant** • All of the listed choices could be part of the contents of an inguinal hernia sac. In a young girl, however, the most likely structure incarcerated in the sac without causing pain would be an ovary. Ovaries can be incarcerated within a hernia sac for long periods of time without producing symptoms. Often the fallopian tube will also be incarcerated in the hernia sac. On the right side, the appendix can be incarcerated in the sac.

**Answers** • 1-D 2-B 3-C

## CASE PRESENTATION

A 1-year-old girl has had progressive weight loss and irritability. She has fully recovered from a prolonged respiratory illness, but does not seem to have regained her appetite and is taking longer naps than usual. She has had no vomiting or diarrhea. A careful physical examination by her pediatrician reveals an immobile solid mass on the right side of her abdomen.

1. The most appropriate radiographic study to order would be:
   A. Abdominal ultrasound
   B. Plain films of the abdomen (KUB)
   C. Upper GI with small-bowel follow-through
   D. Liver-spleen nuclear medicine scan
   E. CT scan of the abdomen and pelvis
2. After review of the imaging studies, a large mass is identified merging with the upper pole of the right kidney. The border between the mass and the right lobe of the liver is indistinct. Calcifications are seen throughout the substance of the mass. Enlarged lymph nodes are seen along the aorta and behind the pancreas. Other laboratory studies that might be helpful in confirming the nature of the mass would include:
   A. Urine collection for vanillylmandelic acid (VMA) and homovanillic acid (HVA)
   B. Serum beta human chorionic gonadotropin (βHCG) levels
   C. 24-hour urine collection for electrolytes
   D. Serum glucose and insulin levels
   E. Serum alpha-fetoprotein levels
3. The most likely diagnosis is
   A. Teratoma (germ cell tumor)
   B. Wilms' tumor (nephroblastoma)
   C. Hepatoblastoma
   D. Neuroblastoma
   E. Pancreatic adenoma
4. A 5-year-old boy presents with a similar physical finding of a large right-sided abdominal mass. Which of the following associated signs or symptoms would point to a diagnosis of Wilms' tumor?
   A. Fever
   B. Unilateral scrotal swelling, "bag of worms"
   C. Decreased urine output
   D. Palpable lymph nodes in the groin or axillary area
   E. Tenderness to palpation over the mass

## COMMENT

**Pediatric abdominal mass evaluation** • The most likely masses in a child of this age would include neuroblastoma, hepatoblastoma, and Wilms' tumor. Ultrasound can localize the mass to the liver, kidney, adrenal, or other location and will also identify cystic areas or calcifications within the substance of the mass. Obstructive renal lesions or cysts within the bowel wall or mesentery may also be identified with ultrasound. CT scan can show similar information with perhaps even more detail, but would require anesthesia or sedation at this age and would not be an ideal first study. Plain films may localize the mass and identify calcifications within the mass, but would not provide as much information as ultrasound. The symptoms do not suggest a GI nature of the mass, so upper GI is not likely to yield a diagnosis. A liver-spleen scan is not a good choice for a screening study and would likely require sedation in most 1-year-old children.

**Laboratory evaluation of pediatric solid tumors** • Location of the mass between the liver and kidney is most consistent with a neuroblastoma. Both hepatoblastoma and Wilms' tumor can be found in this location, but neither is likely to be stippled with calcifications, a finding consistent with neuroblastoma. Neuroblastomas will secrete catecholamines, which are converted into vanillylmandelic acid and homovanillic acid and excreted in the urine. Pancreatic tumors that alter glucose regulation are rare in children and do not present in this location. Both teratoma and hepatoblastoma are associated with elevated serum alpha-fetoprotein levels, but neuroblastoma is the most likely calcified tumor in this area. Lymphadenopathy around the celiac axis (behind the pancreas) is common for neuroblastoma in this location.

**Pediatric solid tumor type** • In addition to the radiographic and laboratory information, the girl's age and symptoms are most consistent with neuroblastoma. Wilms' tumor, the other most common solid tumor in this age group, is rarely symptomatic at presentation. Age of presentation is important in neuroblastoma, because almost all children with neuroblastoma presenting at less than 1 year of age have a good prognosis. Histologic and tumor marker studies determined from biopsy are also extremely important in providing crucial information in neuroblastoma. Differentiation between Wilms' tumor and neuroblastoma is crucial *before* undertaking biopsy, because biopsy of a Wilms' tumor results in tumor spillage and a poorer prognosis. Hepatoblastoma is less likely to present at this age and is usually localized to the liver parenchyma on CT and ultrasound.

**Wilms' tumor** • Wilms' tumor, or nephroblastoma, is usually asymptomatic at presentation. The family member or physician frequently finds the mass incidentally. Fever, fatigue, hypertension, diarrhea, and weight loss are commonly found in neuroblastoma, but rarely in Wilms' tumors. Renal function is usually preserved in Wilms' tumor. Obstruction of the vena cava or the testicular vessels directly may result in a varicocele of the testis that presents as dilated veins within the scrotum (a "bag of worms"). Lymphadenopathy, either within the abdomen or in a palpable nodal basin, is not commonly a feature of Wilms' tumor.

**Answers** • 1-A 2-A 3-D 4-B

## CASE PRESENTATION

A full-term 48-hour-old male infant has not yet passed meconium. A nasogastric tube is placed and returns bilious fluid. The child's abdomen is distended but does not appear to be tender. He is afebrile and his vital signs are normal for an infant this age.

1. Which of the following would be the most appropriate next step in establishing the diagnosis?
   A. Upper gastrointestinal contrast study
   B. Examination of the rectum and perineum
   C. Barium enema
   D. Ultrasound examination of the right upper quadrant
   E. CT scan of the abdomen
2. Your initial evaluation does not establish the diagnosis. An abdominal x-ray reveals multiple uniformly dilated loops of bowel throughout the abdomen. Which of the following is the most likely diagnosis?
   A. Duodenal atresia
   B. Imperforate anus
   C. Hirschsprung's disease
   D. Necrotizing enterocolitis
   E. Intussusception
3. Which of the following would be most definitive in establishing a diagnosis in a *newborn* with distal large-bowel obstruction?
   A. Rectal suction biopsy
   B. Contrast enema
   C. Upper gastrointestinal contrast study
   D. Colonoscopy
   E. Stool examination for fecal leukocytes
4. While awaiting confirmation of your diagnosis, the child develops fever, increasing abdominal distension, abdominal tenderness, and an increasing white blood cell count. The most important step in management is:
   A. Rectal irrigation with isotonic saline solution
   B. Intravenous antibiotic administration
   C. Colonoscopy with large-bowel decompression
   D. Laxative administration
   E. Intravenous promotility agents

## COMMENT

**Initial evaluation of neonatal bowel obstruction** • Meconium normally passes within 24 hours of birth. Failure to pass meconium by 48 hours in a newborn suggests bowel obstruction that will, most likely, require surgical intervention after an appropriate diagnostic evaluation. The differential diagnosis includes Hirschsprung's disease, duodenal or small-bowel atresia, meconium ileus, meconium plug, imperforate anus, and metabolic causes grouped together as small left colon syndrome. Initial evaluation consists of no more than inspection and a simple rectal examination to evaluate the position of the anal opening and rule out imperforate anus. If the anus appears normal on examination, other studies must be considered.

**Diagnosis of neonatal bowel obstruction** • In this case, the presence of air throughout the abdomen eliminates duodenal atresia from the list of possible diagnoses. Duodenal atresia presents with a classic "double bubble" sign on abdominal x-ray evaluation without air in the bowel distal to the ligament of Treitz. On rare occasions, imperforate anus may present with a normal-appearing anus and a rectal stenosis not apparent on examination. This is unusual and would not be the most likely diagnosis. Necrotizing enterocolitis occurs in premature infants rather than in the full-term infant described here. These patients are usually extremely ill, with apparent abdominal pain and tenderness on examination. Intussusception may cause bowel obstruction but commonly occurs in children between 6 months and 1 year of age, although it may occur in older or younger children. While it is difficult, and often impossible, to distinguish small bowel from large bowel on abdominal radiographs in infants, the clinical scenario described here is most consistent with Hirschsprung's disease. Absence of neuroenteric ganglion cells in the wall of the distal large bowel causes an inability for the distal colon to relax, disruption of peristalsis, and failure of colon evacuation. Although usually diagnosed in infancy, this diagnosis should be considered in any child with chronic constipation.

**Diagnosis of Hirschsprung's disease** • Hirschsprung's disease is diagnosed by rectal suction biopsy, which shows an absence of ganglion cells. Contrast enema may show a transition from proximal distended colon to more distal chronically contracted collapsed colon. However, in the neonate, this distinct radiographic finding may not be as apparent as in an older child with a short aganglionic segment and long-standing partial obstruction. Neither upper gastrointestinal contrast study nor stool examination for fecal leukocytes has any significant role in the evaluation of Hirschsprung's disease. Colonoscopy is not an available option in the neonate.

**Hirschsprung's colitis** • Patients with Hirschsprung's disease may develop fulminant colitis with profound sepsis and resultant multiple organ failure. This child shows signs consistent with this diagnosis. Although antibiotic administration is an important component of treatment, the mainstay of therapy is rectal irrigation to evacuate stool trapped proximal to the denervated area. Colonoscopy is not possible in a newborn. Neither laxatives nor promotility agents have any role in the treatment of Hirschsprung's colitis or in uncomplicated Hirschsprung's disease. Treatment is surgical, with excision of the denervated segment and, usually, temporary colostomy. Surgical pull-through of upstream normal bowel to the anus restores continuity of the GI tract with the anal canal and is usually successful in establishing fecal continence.

**Answers** • 1-B 2-C 3-A 4-A

## CASE PRESENTATION

A 3-week-old female infant presents with persistent vomiting. The child is afebrile and her abdomen shows no signs of tenderness. No hernias are present.

1. If the vomitus contains bile, what is the most appropriate initial diagnostic study?
   A. Upper gastrointestinal contrast study
   B. Right upper quadrant ultrasound
   C. Diagnostic laparoscopy
   D. Contrast enema
   E. pH probe study
2. In this patient, bile is *not* present in the vomitus. No abdominal masses are appreciated on examination. What would be the most appropriate initial diagnostic study in this patient?
   A. pH probe study
   B. Radionuclide gastric emptying study
   C. CT scan of the abdomen
   D. Esophagoscopy
   E. Ultrasound of the right upper quadrant of the abdomen
3. Which of the following electrolyte disturbances would be most likely in the patient described?
   A. Increased anion gap metabolic acidosis
   B. Normal anion gap metabolic acidosis
   C. Hypokalemic, hypochloremic metabolic alkalosis
   D. Hyperkalemia with hypernatremia
   E. Hyperkalemia with hypochloremia
4. While awaiting pediatric surgical consultation, which of the following intravenous fluids would be most appropriate?
   A. Lactated Ringer's solution bolus followed by lactated Ringer's solution administered at a maintenance rate
   B. Lactated Ringer's solution bolus followed by D5W 0.45% NSS with 20 mEq KCl/L at a maintenance rate
   C. D5W 0.45% NSS with 20 mEq KCl/L bolus followed by D5W 0.45% NSS with 20 mEq KCl/L at a maintenance rate
   D. D5W 0.45% NSS bolus followed by D5W 0.45% NSS with 40 mEq KCl/L at a maintenance rate
   E. D5W solution at a maintenance rate

## COMMENT

**Bilious vomiting** • Malrotation and intestinal volvulus is the most serious and most critical diagnosis to consider in any young child with bilious vomiting. In this condition, the bowel fails to rotate normally during embryogenesis, leaving the small bowel suspended on a very narrow mesenteric pedicle that can twist, resulting in ischemia and loss of virtually the entire small intestine. Once signs of bowel ischemia develop, it may be too late to salvage the bowel. Thus, diagnosis must be made promptly and before development of abdominal pain or tenderness. Upper gastrointestinal contrast examination will reveal a duodenal sweep that fails to cross the midline and establish a normal position of the ligament of Treitz. Contrast enema may also reveal the diagnosis, but abnormal position of the cecum may occur with normal small-bowel rotation and vice versa. The other studies would not be appropriate to rule out malrotation.

**Nonbilious vomiting** • Nonbilious vomiting suggests obstruction proximal to the sphincter of Oddi. In infants, this is most likely due to pyloric stenosis. Although diagnostic when present, a palpable hypertrophied pyloric "olive" can be difficult to feel in an irritable child. Ultrasound of the right upper quadrant is the most sensitive diagnostic study, with a sensitivity and specificity greater than 95%. In the absence of an experienced pediatric radiologist familiar with the ultrasound findings suggestive of pyloric stenosis, however, an upper gastrointestinal contrast study may be appropriate, although it is less accurate than ultrasound. Narrowing of the pyloric channel results in a "string sign" as contrast passes through the pylorus, and a "shoulder sign" may be present adjacent to the pylorus marking the extent of pyloric muscle thickening. pH probe may be useful to detect esophageal reflux but is not an appropriate first study for the infant with nonbilious vomiting. Esophagoscopy is difficult in young children and is very rarely performed in infants. Although a CT scan may reveal the diagnosis, it is unnecessary and expensive and, in this age group, may require sedation to accomplish. Gastric emptying studies involve leaving a tracer in the stomach for many hours, which is not feasible and may result in aspiration.

**Electrolyte abnormalities due to vomiting** • Patients with intractable vomiting lose both water and electrolytes. Stomach contents are high in hydrochloric acid, so pyloric stenosis patients lose both chloride and hydrogen ions. As the patient becomes more dehydrated, the kidney attempts to preserve intravascular volume by exchanging $Na^+$ in the urine for $K^+$ in the blood, resulting in further $K^+$ loss. $H^+$ losses result in a metabolic alkalosis that can worsen as hypochloremia from $Cl^-$ losses increase and $HCO_3^-$ ions must be reabsorbed from the urine to balance cation absorption. $H^+$ ions are also spilled into the urine in exchange for $Na^+$ ion reabsorbed to preserve blood volume. The result is a hypochloremic, hypokalemic metabolic alkalosis.

**Treatment of vomiting-associated electrolyte disturbances** • Treatment must address both the patient's overall fluid volume status and his or her electrolyte losses. Lactated Ringer's solution is a poor choice in this situation because the infused lactate is converted to $HCO_3^-$, potentially worsening the alkalosis. $K^+$ and $Cl^-$ losses must be replaced. KCl infusion is therefore critical to treatment. Intravenous KCl, however, should not be administered as a rapid bolus. Of the choices listed, only a bolus of D5 0.45% NSS followed by D5 0.45% NSS with 40 mEq KCl/L is appropriate. 0.9% NSS solutions may also be used, and the concentration of KCl can be based on the degree of hypokalemia.

**Answers** • 1-A 2-E 3-C 4-D

## CASE PRESENTATION

A 32-year-old man comes to your emergency department after a fall from a roof. On examination, there is a 9-cm laceration over the right ankle with exposed bone and an obvious deformity. The foot is cool and pulseless, and the patient cannot actively move his toes. Radiographs of his injured ankle are shown (Fig. 1A and 1B).

1. Initial evaluation and management would include:
   A. Administration of intravenous antibiotics and tetanus prophylaxis
   B. Aerobic and anaerobic cultures of the open wounds
   C. Complete examination and application of sterile dressings
   D. All of the above
   E. A and C
2. Which of the following terms accurately describe this injury?
   A. Open, bimalleolar ankle fracture with valgus dislocation
   B. Compound fracture
   C. Spiral fracture of the tibia
   D. All of the above
   E. A and C
3. The most appropriate next step in management is:
   A. Debridement and irrigation of open wounds in the emergency department
   B. An emergent arteriogram of the right lower extremity
   C. Attempted reduction of the fracture
   D. Splinting of the fracture in its current position
   E. Short leg cast application
4. The fracture is reduced. Following treatment in the emergency department, the foot regains its normal color, and sensation and pulses return. Which of the following statements about operative management are true?
   A. Fixation of the fractures with plates and screws should be performed within 6 hours.
   B. Exploration of the posterior tibial artery is not indicated.
   C. Debridement of all nonviable or foreign material as well as pulsatile irrigation of the wounds with saline solution should be performed, and primary closure of open wounds should be avoided.
   D. A and C.
   E. All of the above.

## COMMENT

**Initial evaluation and treatment of open fractures** • In evaluating the patient with an orthopedic injury, it is often easy to focus on the obvious and to overlook potentially life-threatening injuries. The physician must not proceed to the definitive care stage of management without first performing the primary survey, resuscitation, and a complete physical examination to exclude other injuries. Patients with obvious open fractures should have sterile dressings applied to their wounds to avoid further contamination. Antibiotics and appropriate tetanus prophylaxis should be administered early in their evaluation. A first-generation cephalosporin is generally administered for relatively clean or low-energy wounds, with the addition of an aminoglycoside for higher-energy wounds. Penicillin may be added for grossly contaminated wounds that may be contaminated with *Clostridium*. Routine culture of open wounds has poor correlation with established musculoskeletal infections and is not indicated.

**Description of fractures** • Accurate description of an injury is essential. It is important to describe the soft tissue injury (open, closed, contaminated, etc.), the type of fracture (transverse, spiral, oblique, simple, comminuted, etc.), the direction of angulation (anterior, posterior, varus, valgus, etc.), the amount of displacement (nondisplaced, completely displaced, etc.), the bone that is injured, and any associated dislocations. Thus, this injury is most accurately described as an "open, completely displaced, valgus angulated, bimalleolar ankle fracture-dislocation with a syndesmotic disruption and a dysvascular foot. The medial malleolus (tibia) is comminuted and the high lateral malleolar (fibula) fracture is a simple, short-oblique fracture." The term *compound* historically was used to describe open injuries but was often confused with *comminuted* fractures, meaning a fracture with multiple bone fragments. Although still occasionally used, the term *compound* should be avoided.

**Emergent management of open fractures** • In the patient with a nonperfused extremity with a completely displaced fracture or dislocation, reduction of the fracture is an emergency. Appropriate anesthesia should be administered and the fracture reduced. The pulses will usually return and the extremity can then be splinted to maintain the reduction. Emergent arteriograms are not required if normal pulses return with reduction alone. Debridement of devitalized tissue and dilution of the microbial load with pulsatile irrigation is best accomplished in the operating room rather than the emergency room. A circumferential cast is contraindicated in the acute management of this patient.

**Operative management of open fractures** • Following restoration of blood flow, the next most urgent issue is the open injury. This requires debridement and irrigation in the operating room. Delays over 6 hours are associated with limb loss and other complications. Stabilization of the bones to prevent further soft tissue damage is essential. External fixators are often used in grossly contaminated wounds, but implants such as rods, plates, and screws are not contraindicated if the wound is adequately debrided in a timely fashion. Traumatic wounds are closed on a delayed basis to help avoid infection. Since the pulses returned to the patient's foot after reduction of the fracture, there is no need for an arteriogram or exploration in this situation.

**Answers** • 1-E 2-A 3-C 4-E

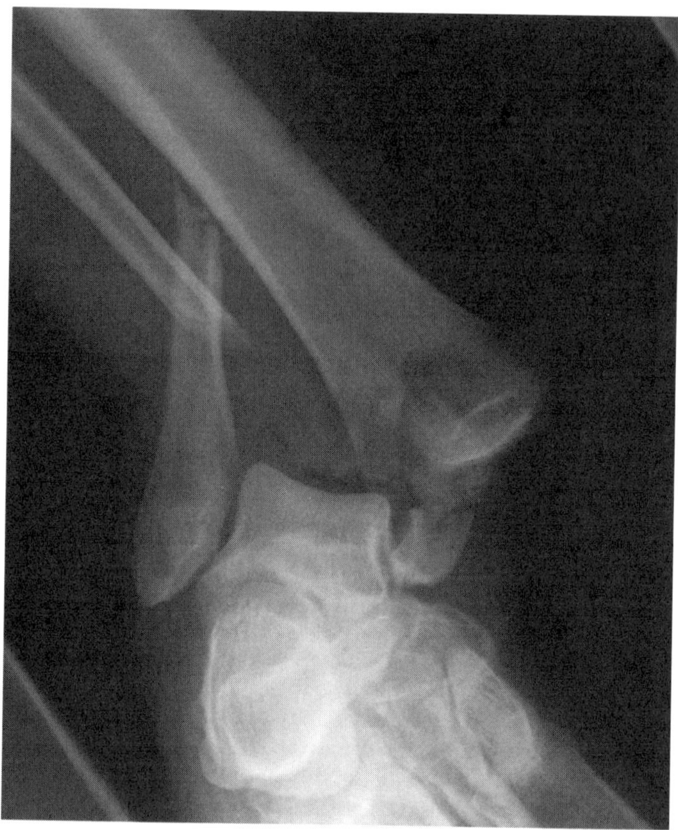

• ***Figure 1A:*** *Image provided by the Medical University of South Carolina, Charleston, South Carolina.*

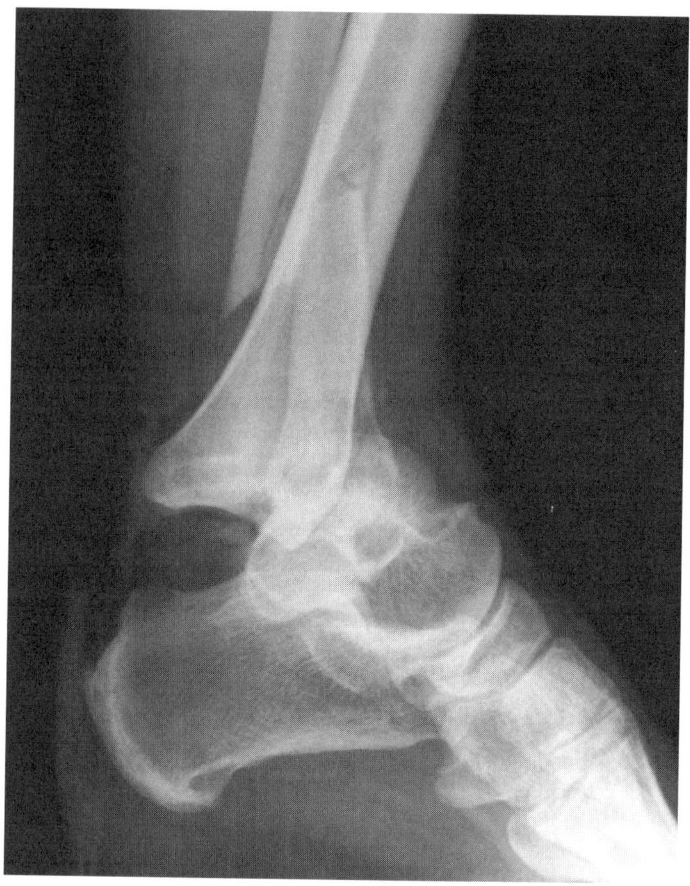

• ***Figure 1B:*** *Image provided by the Medical University of South Carolina, Charleston, South Carolina.*

## CASE PRESENTATION

A 37-year-old man has had 1 year of mild right hip pain that is located in his groin and anterior thigh. It has become much worse in the past month. He denies any trauma to his hip and did not have any hip problems previously. He describes a dull ache with rest and severe pain with weight bearing. Examination of his hip reveals a 15-degree flexion contracture with further forward flexion to 90 degrees. He has no internal rotation and 30 degrees of external rotation. Motion of his hip exacerbates his pain, especially at the extremes of rotation. His radiographs are shown (Fig. 2A and 2B).

1. The most likely diagnosis for his condition is:
   A. Osteonecrosis of the femoral head
   B. Chronic septic arthritis
   C. Primary osteoarthritis
   D. Rheumatoid arthritis
   E. Legg-Calvé-Perthes disease
2. Factors thought to contribute to this condition include:
   A. Alcohol use
   B. Cigarette smoking
   C. Sickle cell disease
   D. All of the above
   E. A and C
3. The best test for early diagnosis of this condition is:
   A. Hip aspiration with cytology and culture
   B. Magnetic resonance imaging (MRI) scan
   C. Hip arthroscopy
   D. Hip arthrogram
   E. Biopsy of femoral head
4. Which of the following are options for treatment?
   A. Total hip arthroplasty
   B. Hip arthrodesis
   C. Core decompression of the femoral head
   D. Conservative measures such as activity modification, nonsteroidal anti-inflammatory medications, and the use of a cane
   E. All of the above

## COMMENT

**Evaluation of hip pain** • Most patients with intra-articular or periarticular pain localize this to the groin or anterior thigh. The complaint may even be of knee pain, especially in the pediatric population where atraumatic knee pain is hip pain until proven otherwise. Duration of the symptoms, exacerbating factors, history of trauma, and the character of the pain are important historical details. Given no prior history of hip problems, Legg-Calvé-Perthes disease can be excluded, since it is a childhood form of osteonecrosis. The acute exacerbation may be consistent with any of the other diagnoses, but is typical of the history given by patients who have osteonecrosis of the femoral head that leads to an area of collapse. The radiographs show areas of sclerosis and lysis in his femoral head, and the weight-bearing portion has become flattened. The joint space remains preserved and there are no significant acetabular changes. This is most consistent with osteonecrosis of the femoral head. There would be loss of the joint space and acetabular changes with any of the other choices, including chronic septic arthritis.

**Causative factors** • Osteonecrosis of the femoral head, also known as aseptic, avascular, or ischemic necrosis, is a common illness in young adults between the ages of 20 and 50. Most often it is the result of trauma, such as femoral neck fractures or hip dislocations, which compromise the blood supply to the femoral head. Osteonecrosis occurs after 10% of hip dislocations or nondisplaced femoral neck fractures and in up to 30% of displaced femoral neck fractures. Nontraumatic osteonecrosis is due to impaired circulation to the femoral head resulting in necrosis and collapse. This may be from external compression of vessels, thrombosis, or embolization. It is also often associated with sickle cell disease or certain coagulopathies. Excessive alcohol use or high doses of corticosteroids are associated with 70% of cases of nontraumatic osteonecrosis, but the exact mechanism is poorly understood. Although there is a vascular mechanism, there is no clear association with tobacco use.

**Diagnosis** • Diagnosis is often difficult, because radiographic signs such as areas of sclerosis or lucency do not appear for the first several months. If diagnosed before collapse of the femoral head, treatment results are much better. MRI is highly sensitive and specific and is the best diagnostic test for the early stages of osteonecrosis. The other tests listed do not have a role in the diagnosis of this condition.

**Treatment** • Treatment depends on the amount of collapse and secondary arthritis. Conservative measures, although usually ineffective, can be employed in patients who are not ready for surgical intervention. Decompression of the ischemic area (core decompression) relieves the increased intraosseous pressure in the femoral head and allows for vascular ingrowth and new bone formation and is effective in about 65% of patients. The addition of a vascularized bone graft raises the success rate to 80% in patients without collapse, but adds donor site morbidity. Arthrodesis of the hip is a durable option, but it is often difficult to achieve fusion if there is extensive necrosis, and patients are often reluctant to accept a fused hip. Total hip arthroplasty and resurfacing arthroplasty have both had disappointing results in the past. Newer devices and techniques, however, have demonstrated improved results and prosthetic replacement is rapidly becoming the treatment of choice for osteonecrosis with collapse. Since there is no deformity on the acetabular side, there is little role for a periacetabular osteotomy in this patient.

**Answers** • 1-A 2-E 3-B 4-E

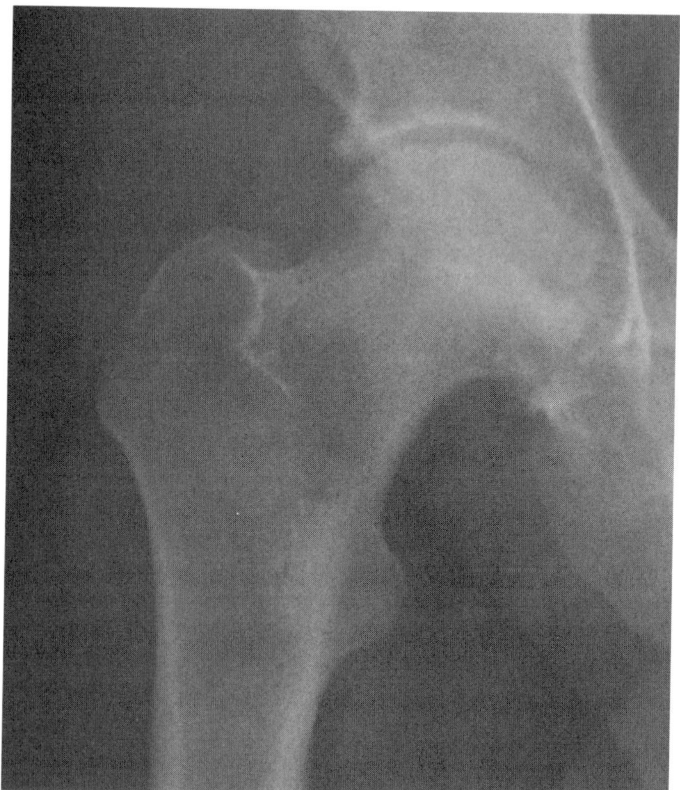

• ***Figure 2A:*** *Image provided by the Medical University of South Carolina, Charleston, South Carolina.*

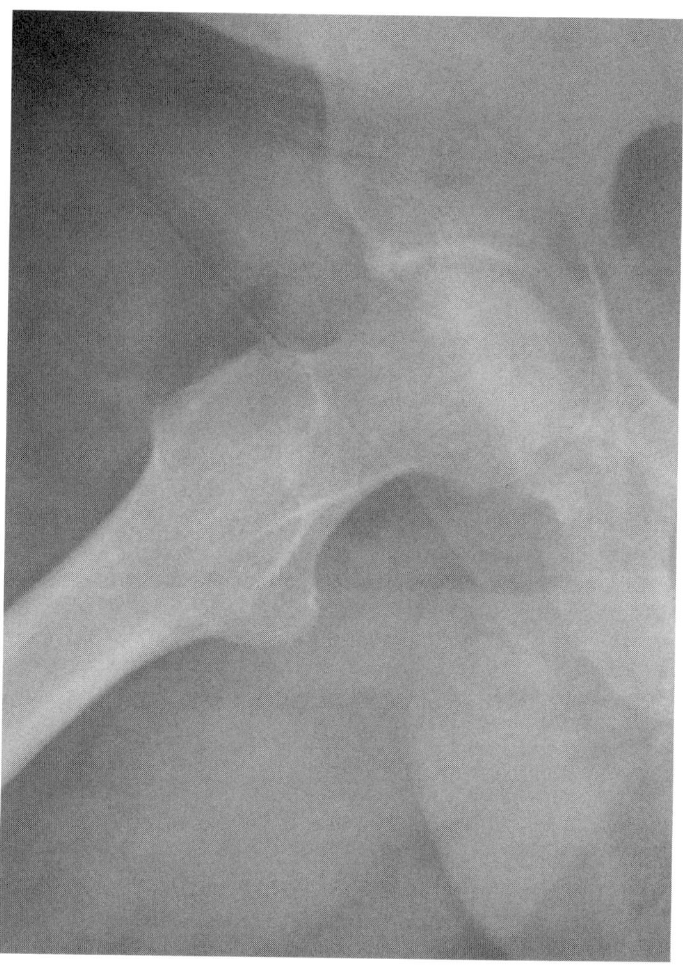

• ***Figure 2B:*** *Image provided by the Medical University of South Carolina, Charleston, South Carolina.*

## CASE PRESENTATION

A healthy, active, 50-year-old patient who underwent a total hip arthroplasty (THA) and did well for 10 years returns complaining of a recent onset of groin pain. His erythrocyte sedimentation rate is slightly elevated and his C-reactive protein is normal. The radiograph obtained is shown (Fig. 3).

1. The most likely reason for his pain is:
   A. Infection of his THA
   B. Osteolysis from polyethylene wear debris
   C. Loosening of the prosthetic components
   D. Metastatic cancer
   E. Trochanteric bursitis
2. The best treatment option is:
   A. 6 weeks of intravenous antibiotic therapy
   B. Revision arthroplasty with bone grafting
   C. Injection of corticosteroids into the joint space
   D. Rest for 6 weeks followed by physical therapy
   E. Oral nonsteroidal anti-inflammatory agents
3. Two days after having hip surgery, the patient suddenly develops tachypnea. $Pao_2$ is slightly decreased. Breath sounds are equal bilaterally. A chest radiograph is unremarkable. Which of the following is the most likely diagnosis?
   A. Adult respiratory distress syndrome (ARDS)
   B. Congestive heart failure
   C. Pneumonia
   D. Pulmonary embolus
   E. Lobar atelectasis
4. Which of the following tests would be most likely to reveal the diagnosis above?
   A. Electrocardiogram
   B. CT scan of the chest with contrast bolus
   C. Ventilation/perfusion scan
   D. Bronchoscopy
   E. Insertion of Swan-Ganz catheter
5. Which of the following treatments is most appropriate?
   A. Aggressive diuresis
   B. Intubation and subsequent bronchoscopy
   C. Immediate initiation of warfarin therapy
   D. Thrombolytic agents
   E. None of the above

## COMMENT

**Failed total hip arthroplasty** • One of the most common reasons for delayed failure of an ingrown total hip arthroplasty is osteolysis secondary to polyethylene wear debris. It is estimated that up to 500,000 submicron particles of polyethylene are generated with each step during normal gait. As the body attempts to eliminate this debris, macrophages release prostaglandins, interleukins, and tumor necrosis factor, leading to resorption of surrounding bone known as osteolysis. This is demonstrated in the radiograph as lytic defects in the proximal femur and large defects in the superior acetabulum and medial wall. The worn polyethylene component is demonstrated by the eccentricity of the femoral head in the acetabulum. Despite the osteolysis, the components remain well fixed. Although infection or metastatic disease are possibilities, the most likely choice is osteolysis.

**Treatment for failed total hip arthroplasty** • These radiographs demonstrate catastrophic wear of the polyethylene and severe osteolysis. Revision surgery to correct the progressively worsening problem is essential. If left untreated, complete failure of the polyethylene with resultant metal-on-metal wear is inevitable. Because infection is unlikely with a normal C-reactive protein, antibiotic treatment is not indicated. This patient had bone grafting of the large femoral and acetabular defects and replacement of the metal acetabular shell, polyethylene liner, and femoral head.

**Postoperative pulmonary complications** • All of the complications listed are seen in hospitalized patients. Pneumonia, lobar atelectasis, adult respiratory distress syndrome, pulmonary congestion, and pneumothorax would be apparent on chest radiographs (and would be associated with an abnormal physical exam). ARDS causes profound hypoxemia. This patient's mild hypoxemia and the clinical setting are consistent with small pulmonary embolus.

**Diagnosis of pulmonary embolus** • Pulmonary angiography remains the gold standard for diagnosis of pulmonary embolus. While a high-probability ventilation/perfusion (V/Q) scan reliably identifies pulmonary emboli, low- or moderate-probability scans can miss significant emboli. Rapid spiral CT scan of the chest during a contrast bolus can reliably detect small pulmonary emboli without the risks of pulmonary angiography.

**Treatment of pulmonary embolus** • Clot lysis is indicated in cases of severe pulmonary embolus with hemodynamic instability, but not for small emboli, as in this case (plus, the recent surgery is a contraindication). Warfarin therapy should be considered for long-term anticoagulation; however, its slow onset of action makes it unsuitable for immediate use. Treatment options for acute pulmonary embolism include heparin or low-molecular-weight heparin. If those are contraindicated, the next step is interruption of the vena cava with intravascular filter placement. Neither diuresis nor bronchoscopy has any role in the treatment of pulmonary embolism.

**Answers** • 1-B 2-B 3-D 4-B 5-E

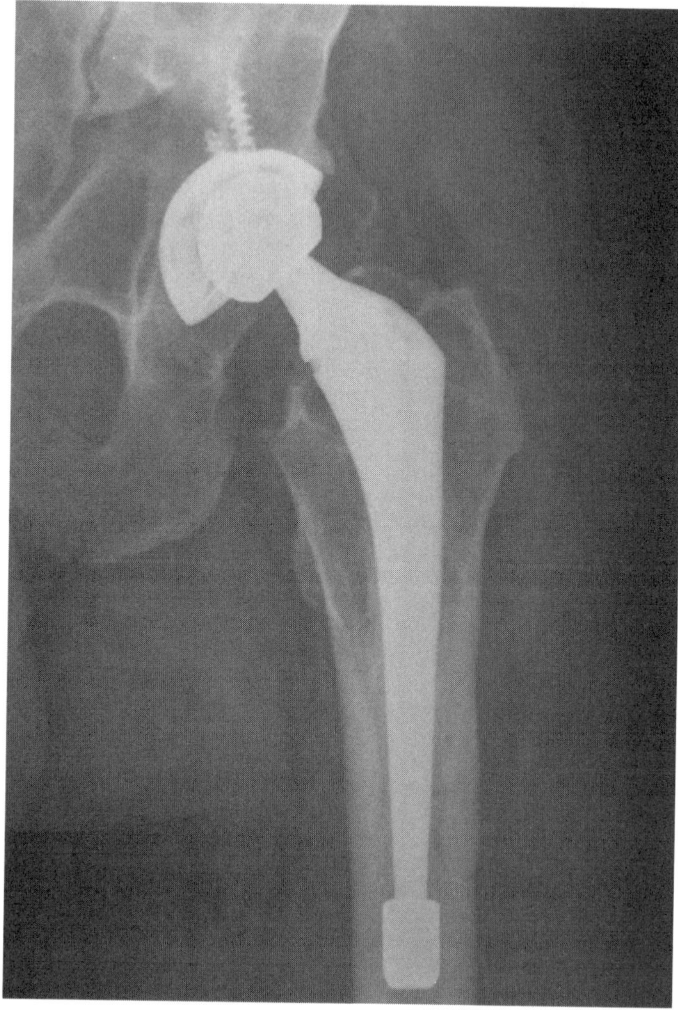

• ***Figure 3:*** *Image provided by the Medical University of South Carolina, Charleston, South Carolina.*

## CASE PRESENTATION

A healthy 15-year-old boy injures his knee while playing basketball and sustains the injury shown (Fig. 4A and 4B).

1. Which portion of the bone is injured?
   A. Metaphysis
   B. Physis
   C. Epiphysis
   D. Apophysis
   E. All of the above
2. The portion of the fracture that traverses the growth plate usually goes mostly through which zone?
   A. Reserve (resting) zone
   B. Proliferative zone
   C. Hypertrophic (maturation, degenerative, and provisional calcification) zone
   D. None of the above
   E. All of the above
3. The most likely mechanism of injury is:
   A. Varus stress
   B. Valgus stress
   C. Torsional stress
   D. Forced flexion against resistance
   E. None of the above

## COMMENT

**Definitions and bone growth** • Bones form and grow by either intramembranous or enchondral ossification. Intramembranous ossification is responsible for the formation of flat bones (e.g., pelvis, skull). Enchondral ossification occurs in the formation of long bones (e.g., femur, radius). In children, long bones have several distinct regions. The diaphysis is the central shaft of a long bone. The metaphysis is the flared region, consisting largely of cancellous bone, at either end of the shaft but central to the growth plate. The physis is the cartilaginous growth plate itself. The epiphysis is a secondary ossification center at either end of the bone. An apophysis is an outgrowth that is responsible for formation of various tuberosities, tubercles, and trochanters. The fracture shown involves the central epiphysis, the physis, the tubercle apophysis, and the posterior metaphysis. The diaphysis is not involved in this fracture.

**Physeal zones** • The physis can be divided into three zones. The *reserve zone* is closest to the epiphysis. The chondrocytes are spherical and widely dispersed. In the *proliferative zone,* the chondrocytes proliferate and become flattened and longitudinally aligned. This proliferation and reorientation, combined with continued matrix production, creates longitudinal growth. The *hypertrophic zone* is subdivided into the maturation zone, degenerative zone, and zone of provisional calcification. Chondrocytes increase in size and die. Osteoblasts use the cartilage scaffolding to form bone. Mineralization occurs at the portion of the hypertrophic zone closest to the metaphysis. Physeal fractures usually occur through the hypertrophic zone, in the zone of provisional calcification, and often extend into the metaphysis (Salter-Harris types I and II), thus leaving the resting and proliferative zones uninjured. This is why growth arrest or physeal bar formation is rare in the Salter-Harris (SH) I and II fractures, but more common in the III and IV fractures, which traverse the hypertrophic zone and extend into the resting and proliferative zones.

**Mechanism** • By examining the angulation of the fracture and the direction of displacement, the treating physician can often understand the mechanism of injury. This is important to determine prior to planning any reduction maneuvers or fracture stabilization. In this fracture, there is little varus or valgus angulation to suggest a varus or valgus load. Torsional stresses usually produce spiral fractures. The fracture shown is the result of the extremely high contractile force of the extensor mechanism against resistance. The tibial tubercle was displaced through its apophysis, and the forces extended proximally, through the physis and epiphysis, into the knee joint (an SH type III fracture). There was a secondary fracture extending from the joint through the epiphysis, physis, and posterior metaphysis (an SH type IV fracture), which is a rare variant of this injury.

**Answers** • 1-E 2-C 3-D

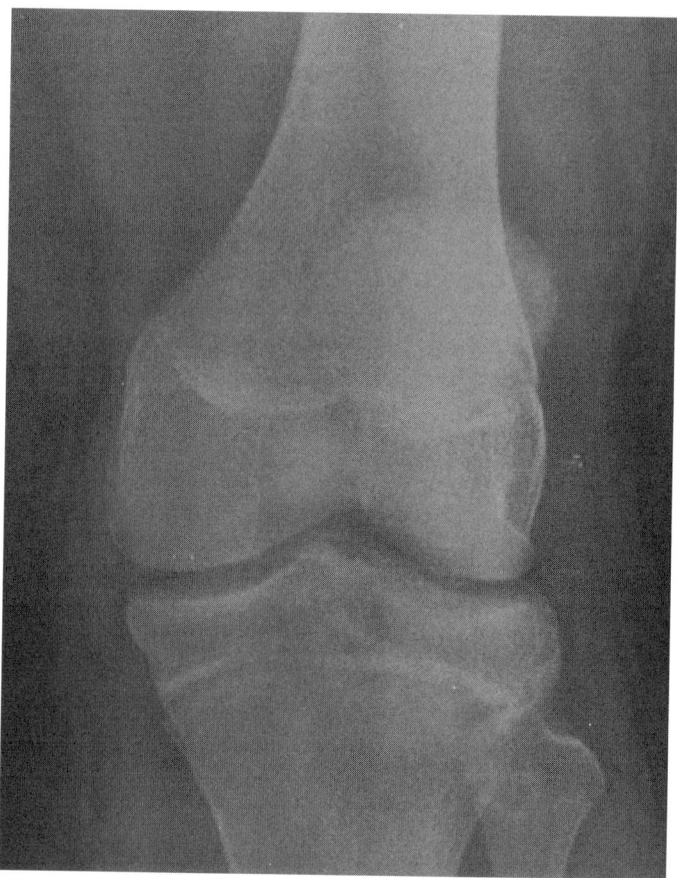

• ***Figure 4A:*** *Image provided by the Medical University of South Carolina, Charleston, South Carolina.*

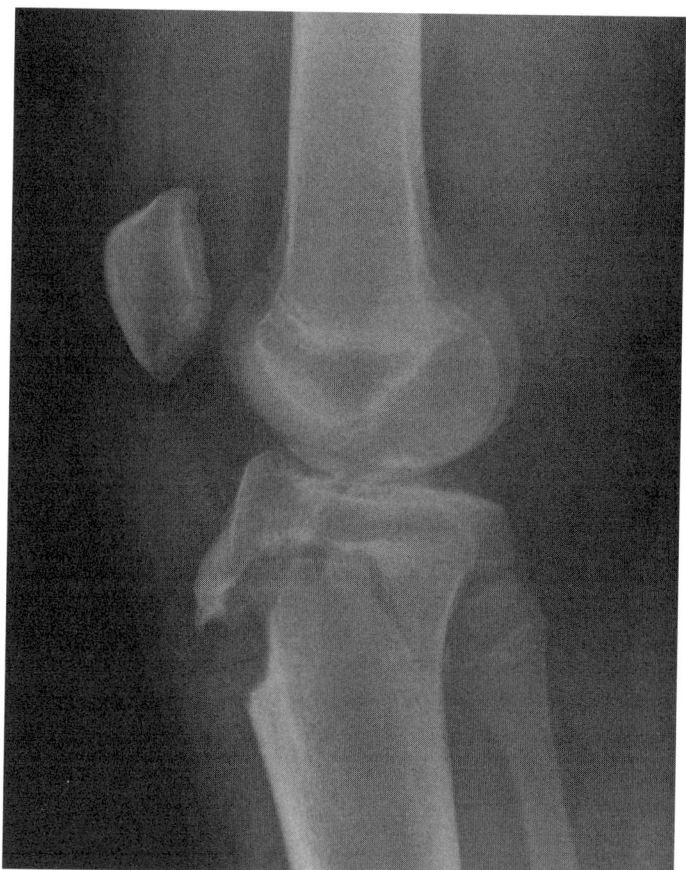

• ***Figure 4B:*** *Image provided by the Medical University of South Carolina, Charleston, South Carolina.*

## CASE PRESENTATION

A 65-year-old man is referred for evaluation of an elevated prostate-specific antigen (PSA). On routine evaluation, the level was found to be 9.5 ng/mL. A review of his medical record indicates the level was 2.5 ng/mL 14 months earlier. The patient denies any hematuria, dysuria, frequency, or urgency. He does report nocturia once per night. On exam there is a small nodular prostate.

1. Which of the following may cause an elevated PSA?
   A. Acute prostatitis
   B. Recent Foley catheter
   C. Prostate infarct
   D. Bladder cancer
   E. A, B, and C
2. Possibly effective treatment options for patients with localized prostate cancer may include:
   A. Radical prostatectomy
   B. Chemotherapy
   C. Radiation therapy
   D. A and C
   E. A, B, and C
3. The most likely site of extranodal spread for prostate cancer is:
   A. Bone
   B. Liver
   C. Lung
   D. Brain
   E. Kidney
4. With respect to prostate cancer, which of the following is true?
   A. A serum PSA level of greater than 4.0 ng/mL is diagnostic of prostate cancer.
   B. Prostate cancer is the most common non-skin cancer in men.
   C. Prostate cancer is the most common cause of cancer deaths in men.
   D. African American and white men have similar incidences of prostate cancer.
   E. The American Cancer Society recommends all men begin prostate cancer screening at age 40.

## COMMENT

**Prostate-specific antigen** • Prostate-specific antigen (PSA) is a glycoprotein produced by prostate epithelial cells. The role that PSA plays in fertility is not entirely clear, but it does act to hydrolyze the coagulum of the ejaculate. Any insult to the prostate epithelial cells can cause a rise in serum PSA. Acute prostatitis is an inflammatory process usually caused by bacterial infection. Patients may present with fevers, back pain, perineal pain, varying degrees of urinary retention, and general malaise. Serum PSA is not used in the diagnosis, but acute prostatitis will elevate the PSA level. Prostate infarct results from occlusion of small blood vessels within the prostate. Symptoms include urinary retention and a tender, enlarged prostate. Instrumentation, including recent catheterization, can disrupt the epithelial cells and result in transient rises in PSA. Prostate cancer results in disruption of the epithelial cells, allowing for PSA levels to rise. Interestingly, only 25% of patients with a PSA between 4.0 ng/mL and 10.0 ng/mL will have prostate cancer found on biopsy. Bladder cancer does not damage the prostate epithelial cells and thus does not elevate the PSA.

**Treatment of prostate cancer** • Localized prostate cancer is curable with surgical therapy, external beam radiotherapy, and interstitial radiation therapy (brachytherapy). Cryotherapy is becoming a standard method of treatment, though long-term results are less certain than other standard therapies. To date there is no effective chemotherapy for either localized or metastatic prostate cancer. Prostate cancer is an androgen-sensitive malignancy; therefore, hormone ablation therapy is widely used for metastatic disease. While not curative, it does slow the progression of the disease.

**Metastatic spread of prostate cancer** • The spread of prostate cancer is first to the pelvic lymph nodes. Extranodal spread typically is to the axial skeleton. In contrast to most metastatic disease to bone, prostate cancer results in blastic bone lesions. Early symptoms of metastatic prostate cancer include bone pain and pathologic fractures. Spread to the viscera and brain is rare and occurs late in the progression of the disease.

**Prostate cancer screening** • An elevated serum PSA is not diagnostic of prostate cancer PSA is used as a screening test that, along with digital rectal examination, suggests which men are at high risk for the disease and thus should have prostate biopsy. Prostate cancer is the most common non-skin cancer found in men. It is estimated that 41% of all non-skin cancer diagnoses made yearly in males are prostate cancer. Lung cancer remains the leading cause of cancer deaths in men, with prostate cancer second. African American men have an increased risk for prostate cancer and have higher death rates than white men. The American Cancer Society recommends that men with a life expectancy greater than 10 years be offered prostate cancer screening with yearly digital rectal exam and PSA beginning at age 50. Screening for African American men and men with a first-degree relative with prostate cancer should be offered beginning at age 45.

**Answers** • 1-E 2-D 3-A 4-B

## CASE PRESENTATION

A 42-year-old woman has an abdominal ultrasound for right upper quadrant pain. Mention is made of a well-defined left lower pole renal mass. The mass is described as being oval, thin walled, without internal echoes, and with posterior acoustic enhancement. Size measurements are given as 3 cm by 4 cm. No other abnormalities are noted and she has no family history of kidney disease.

1. The most likely diagnosis in this patient is:
   - A. Renal cell carcinoma
   - B. Angiomyolipoma
   - C. Renal cyst
   - D. Oncocytoma
   - E. Adult polycystic kidney disease
2. The most logical next step is:
   - A. CT scan of the abdomen with and without IV contrast
   - B. Intravenous pyelogram (IVP)
   - C. Repeat ultrasound in 6 months
   - D. No further follow-up
   - E. Surgical excision of the mass
3. Adult polycystic kidney disease may be accompanied by:
   - A. Berry aneurysms of the circle of Willis
   - B. Cerebellar hemangioblastomas
   - C. Hepatic cyst, hypertension, and renal failure
   - D. All of the above
   - E. A and C

## COMMENT

**Causes of renal masses** • Incidental renal masses are often found during evaluation for other diseases. In this case the patient was having ultrasound for presumed cholelithiasis. The mass in question is described as a well-defined, thin-walled anechoic mass with posterior acoustic shadowing. It meets all requirements for a simple cyst. Benign renal cyst is the most commonly found renal mass. Renal cell carcinomas, angiomyolipomas, and oncocytomas are all solid lesions, although they may have a cystic component. On ultrasound imaging, they would not show all of the features of a cyst. Any lesion that does not clearly meet all the criteria for a simple cyst must be considered a solid lesion. Solid masses detected on ultrasound are most commonly renal cell carcinoma. Adult polycystic kidney disease is an autosomal dominant disease, and there is usually a family history. On ultrasound, multiple cysts are present in both kidneys.

**Evaluation of renal mass** • The mass in question is a simple cyst and thus no further evaluation is needed. If the radiographic criteria of a simple cyst were not met, the logical next step would be CT scan. With the use of pre- and postcontrast imaging, the presence of a solid component can be determined. More than 90% of solid renal tumors are malignant; therefore, the determination of cystic versus solid mass is very important. Repeat ultrasound is not indicated for simple cyst. Surgical excision is not indicated for a simple cyst.

**Adult polycystic kidney disease** • Adult polycystic kidney disease is an autosomal dominant disorder that affects multiple organ systems. Symptoms usually first occur in the fourth to sixth decade of life with hypertension, hematuria, abdominal pain, renal colic, and progressive renal insufficiency. Other organ systems are affected. Nonrenal findings include berry aneurysms in 10% to 40% of patients, hepatic cyst in up to 60% of patients, and diverticular disease. (Note that cerebellar hemangioblastomas; retinal angiomas; cysts of the pancreas, kidney, and epididymis; pheochromocytomas; and renal cell carcinomas constitute von Hippel-Lindau disease, which is also autosomal dominant.)

**Answers** • 1-C 2-D 3-E

## CASE PRESENTATION

A 16-year-old boy presents with a 2-day history of painful scrotal swelling. His pain started during the night and was severe enough to wake him. Nonsteroidal anti-inflammatory medications have not controlled the pain. Physical examination shows a healthy-appearing male in moderate distress. The right hemiscrotum is painful and swollen, with a high-riding testicle. The contralateral testicle is normal. Urine analysis is normal.

1. What is the next step?
   - A. Doppler ultrasound of the scrotum
   - B. Treatment with antibiotics
   - C. Radical orchiectomy
   - D. Scrotal exploration
   - E. CT scan of the abdomen
2. With regard to scrotal masses, which of the following is true?
   - A. Orchitis is the most common cause of a scrotal mass.
   - B. Testicular cancer is the most common cause of a scrotal mass.
   - C. Varicoceles are the most common cause of a scrotal mass.
   - D. Hydroceles are the most common cause of a scrotal mass.
   - E. Testicular cancer is a rare form of cancer in young males.
3. With regard to testicular cancer, which of the following is true?
   - A. Testicular cancer is the most common malignancy of young males.
   - B. African American males are affected more commonly than are white males.
   - C. The first site of spread is to the retroperitoneal lymph nodes.
   - D. Alpha-fetoprotein (AFP) is elevated in both non-seminoma and seminoma.
   - E. Beta human chorionic gonadotropin (β-hCG) is elevated in the majority of patients with seminoma.

## COMMENT

**Acute scrotal pain** • The most common diagnosis for a 16-year-old boy with acute scrotal pain and a normal urinalysis is testicular torsion. This constitutes a urologic emergency. With the given history, the most logical step would be scrotal exploration with orchiopexy of the affected testicle, if viable, and orchiopexy of the contralateral testicle. Time is of utmost importance, with testicular salvage rates reduced after 4 hours. Doppler ultrasound is only utilized when there is a low index of suspicion for torsion. Imaging should never delay surgical exploration when one suspects that torsion is present. Contralateral orchiopexy is always performed because the "bell clapper" deformity that predisposes to torsion occurs bilaterally. With proper repair, there is no chance of repeat torsion. Radical orchiectomy is removal of the testes and cord structures to the level of the internal inguinal ring, and is utilized in the treatment of testicular cancer. There is no indication of infection, so treatment with antibiotics would be inappropriate.

**Scrotal masses:** • Hydrocele is the most common scrotal mass. It results from fluid collection between the tunica vaginalis and the testes. Hydroceles may be congenital or may result from trauma, previous surgery, or malignancy. The sudden onset of a hydrocele should raise suspicion of cancer. Varicoceles result from an engorgement of the venous drainage of the testes. Due to anatomic variances, varicoceles occur on the left about 95% of the time. Right-sided varicoceles are suggestive of retroperitoneal disease. Orchitis is infection of the testes. It presents as painful swelling of the testes with signs of urinary tract infection. Malignancy must be considered, but careful history and physical exam will lead to the correct diagnosis. Testicular cancer is the most common intratesticular mass.

**Testicular cancer** • Testicular cancer is the most common solid tumor of men between the ages of 20 and 34, but hematologic malignancies remain the most common malignancies in that age group. African American men are affected only about one-third as often as white men. Common presenting symptoms include a testicular mass with or without testicular pain, testicular pain alone, infertility, acute onset of a hydrocele, and metastatic lesions with an unknown primary in a young man. The site of lymphatic spread follows the testicular blood supply and thus is to the retroperitoneal lymph nodes rather than the lymph nodes of the groin region. Right-sided tumors tend to spread to the paracaval and intra-aortocaval nodes, whereas left-sided tumors tend to be para-aortic.

Testicular cancer is divided into two broad categories, seminoma and non-seminoma. Seminoma is slightly more common and occurs in an older population. Non-seminoma includes choriocarcinoma, yolk sac tumors, embryonal carcinoma, and teratocarcinoma. Non-seminoma may produce both β-hCG and AFP. These are important markers in the diagnosis and continued management of testicular cancer patients. Seminoma will produce β-hCG about 10% of the time. They do not produce AFP. An elevated AFP excludes the diagnosis of seminoma. (This level of detail will probably not be tested on the boards.) Overall, testicular cancers are highly curable, with a 5-year survival of greater than 90%. Treatment involves a multimodal approach that includes surgery, chemotherapy, and radiation therapy.

**Answers** • 1-D 2-D 3-C

## CASE PRESENTATION

A 50-year-old man has had gradually progressive dyspnea on exertion and fatigue. On examination, a grade II/VI systolic murmur at the apex and radiating to the axilla is noted. He also has an S3 gallop and an irregular cardiac rhythm. Echocardiography reveals severe mitral regurgitation.

1. What is the most likely cause of this patient's mitral regurgitation?
   A. Mitral valve prolapse
   B. Ischemia
   C. Rheumatic heart disease
   D. Endocarditis
   E. A history of untreated syphilis
2. The best surgical treatment for mitral valve prolapse is:
   A. Mitral valve repair
   B. Mechanical valve replacement with a tilting disc prosthesis
   C. Replacement with porcine valve prosthesis
   D. Replacement with human tissue valve prosthesis
   E. Replacement with pericardial valve prosthesis
3. Which of the following requires long-term anticoagulation?
   A. Mitral valve annuloplasty
   B. Mitral valve repair
   C. Mitral valve replacement with mechanical prosthesis
   D. Mitral valve replacement with bioprosthesis (e.g., porcine pericardial valve)
   E. All of the above
4. In which of the following patients with severe mitral regurgitation is medical therapy alone most appropriate?
   A. Asymptomatic patient with a normal ejection fraction, a nondilated ventricle, atrial fibrillation, and in whom valve repair appears technically feasible
   B. Symptomatic patient with an ejection fraction less than 25% in whom valve repair does not appear technically feasible
   C. Asymptomatic patient with a normal ejection fraction, a nondilated ventricle, pulmonary hypertension, and in whom valve repair appears technically feasible
   D. Symptomatic patient with an ejection fraction greater than 45% in whom valve repair appears technically feasible
   E. Asymptomatic patient with a 55% ejection fraction, a dilated ventricle, pulmonary hypertension, and in whom valve repair does not appear technically feasible

## COMMENT

**Etiology of mitral regurgitation** • The most common cause of severe mitral regurgitation is mitral valve prolapse (at least 50% of cases needing surgery). Other causes include ischemia (25%), rheumatic heart disease (10% to 15%), and endocarditis (10%). Syphilis is not associated with mitral regurgitation but may be associated with aortic regurgitation and thoracic aortic aneurysm formation (a rare illness in the developed world).

**Repair options** • Simple repair of the valve is preferable to replacement with a prosthetic valve. This eliminates the need for anticoagulation and its inherent risk of bleeding. Repair also preserves the subvalvular apparatus that supports the left ventricle wall, maintaining the conical shape of the ventricle and thus better preserving left ventricular function (the papillary muscles contribute to ejection fraction). Artificial valves also carry an increased risk of endocarditis. Unfortunately, repair is not always possible, especially in patients with rheumatic heart disease or endocarditis.

**Anticoagulation after valve surgery** • Use of mechanical valves requires anticoagulation. Bioprosthetic valves do not have this requirement. However, currently available bioprosthetic valves have a shorter useful life than mechanical valves. The risk of anticoagulation must be balanced against the need for replacement. Neither annuloplasty or direct valve repair requires anticoagulation.

**Indications for surgery** • In patients with symptomatic severe mitral regurgitation, surgical treatment is appropriate except for those with severe left ventricular dysfunction. In asymptomatic patients, surgery should be performed before the onset of irreversible ventricular dysfunction. However, it can be difficult to identify the onset of early ventricular dysfunction. Currently, left ventricular end systolic dimension and ejection fraction are used to monitor ventricular performance and identify patients with severe mitral regurgitation that would benefit from valve replacement. An ejection fraction less than 60% or a dilated ventricle with an end systolic dimension greater than 45 mm are considered indicators of early systolic dysfunction, especially if progressive, and would warrant consideration for operative repair. Other factors that may be considered indications for surgery include new atrial fibrillation, development of pulmonary hypertension, and the potential repairability of the valve. Patients with potentially repairable valves may be treated with surgery earlier than those who will require valve replacement.

Some of these indications are subject to debate. But all agree that severe left ventricular dysfunction is a contraindication to surgical correction of mitral regurgitation.

**Answers** • 1-A 2-A 3-C 4-B

## CASE PRESENTATION

A 72-year-old woman with a history of hypertension suffered an anterior myocardial infarction 4 days ago. Her blood pressure has been stable for 3 days. She does not require supplemental oxygen. She suddenly develops a full feeling in her chest, becomes short of breath, hypotensive, and tachycardic. Physical examination reveals a loud systolic murmur that was not present at the time of admission.

1. Of the following, which is most likely?
   A. Dressler's syndrome (postinfarction pericarditis)
   B. Ascending aortic dissection
   C. Free rupture of the posterolateral left ventricular wall
   D. Atrial septal defect
   E. Acute mitral regurgitation from papillary muscle rupture
2. Which of these diagnostic studies is most likely to reveal the cause for the patient's deterioration?
   A. Coronary angiography
   B. Signal-averaged electrocardiography
   C. Echocardiography
   D. CT scan of the chest
   E. Magnetic resonance angiography
3. A Swan-Ganz catheter reveals higher oxygen saturations in the pulmonary artery than in the right atrium (a "step up"). The best management plan is:
   A. Delayed repair to allow fibrosis of the edge of the defect to ensure secure suture placement
   B. Pharmacologic afterload reduction
   C. Placement of an intra-aortic balloon pump and emergency operative repair
   D. High-dose inotropic support
   E. Vigorous diuresis
4. Which of the following would be the most appropriate method of surgical management of this patient?
   A. Mitral valve ring annuloplasty
   B. Valve replacement with an artificial valve
   C. Human tissue valve replacement
   D. Primary repair of the defect
   E. Closure of the defect with a Dacron patch

## COMMENT

**Mechanical complications of myocardial infarction** • Ventricular septal rupture (causing ventriculoseptal defect) and acute mitral regurgitation from papillary muscle rupture require immediate surgical intervention. Both cause a new and loud systolic murmur after myocardial infarction (MI), and it is not possible to distinguish between them with physical exam. Rupture of the free wall of the ventricle does not cause a murmur, and death from tamponade is usually sudden. Atrial septal defect is a congenital condition and is not a complication of acute myocardial infarction. Cardiogenic shock may also be considered a "mechanical" complication of MI, and can be treated with urgent revascularization (usually with angioplasty).

Acute ventriculoseptal defect (VSD) and mitral regurgitation may result in pulmonary edema and cardiogenic shock. Dressler's syndrome, or postinfarction pericarditis, causes chest pain, fever, friction rub, dyspnea, malaise, and occasionally a pericardial effusion large enough to produce symptoms of pericardial tamponade. Aortic dissection is not a complication of myocardial infarction.

**Diagnostic evaluation** • Echocardiography is the procedure of choice for evaluation of new murmurs. Although not needed for initial diagnosis, coronary angiography is performed in relatively stable patients to allow the surgeon to bypass blocked coronary arteries at the time of repair of the acute lesion. Signal-averaged echocardiography is used to predict the risk of ventricular arrhythmias but has no role in evaluation of this patient's deterioration.

**Management** • A step up in hemoglobin oxygen saturation is diagnostic of a left-to-right intracardiac shunt (in this case, VSD; a step up is also seen with atrial septal defect). Catecholamine support of blood pressure, afterload reduction, and diuresis may be needed as supportive care, but immediate surgical repair is the definitive therapy. Intra-aortic balloon counterpulsation decreases afterload while improving both systemic and coronary artery perfusion, and is a useful bridge to surgery.

**Repair** • Based on the "step up" in hemoglobin saturation, our patient has a VSD and needs closure of the defect. An occasional patient with acute mitral regurgitation can have valve repair, but most need replacement.

**Answers** • 1-E 2-C 3-C 4-E

## CASE PRESENTATION

A 45-year-old man presents to the emergency department with sudden onset of severe tearing chest pain. The pain was at maximum severity at its onset. His electrocardiogram is normal. His past medical history is significant for hypertension and an ankle fracture 15 years previously.

1. Which test would you do first?
   A. Coronary angiography
   B. Magnetic resonance imaging (MRI) of the chest
   C. Computed tomographic (CT) angiography of the chest
   D. Transthoracic echocardiogram
   E. Aortogram
2. Evaluation reveals an aortic dissection involving the ascending aorta but not involving the aortic arch or descending aorta. What is the best management of this patient?
   A. Urgent surgery with replacement of the ascending aorta
   B. Intra-aortic balloon counterpulsation until surgery can be performed
   C. Beta blockade and afterload reduction alone
   D. Beta blockade and afterload reduction with delayed repair to allow fibrosis of the aortic wall to ensure secure suture placement
   E. Heparinization to prevent clotting within the false lumen
3. While awaiting the arrival of the consulting surgeon, the patient becomes hypotensive, dyspneic, plethoric, and has distended neck veins. Which of the following most likely explains his deterioration?
   A. Acute aortic valve regurgitation
   B. Distal extension of the dissection to involve the aortic arch and carotid arteries
   C. Dissection into a coronary artery with occlusion leading to acute myocardial infarction and congestive heart failure
   D. Rupture into the pericardium with pericardial tamponade
   E. Rupture into the right pleural cavity with massive right hemothorax
4. Which of the following is a risk factor for development of this condition?
   A. Elevated serum cholesterol levels
   B. A history of untreated syphilis
   C. Hypertension
   D. A 30-pack-year smoking history
   E. Presence of an abdominal aortic aneurysm

## COMMENT

**Diagnosis of aortic dissection** • The pain of acute dissection is as bad at its onset as it ever gets (pain at the onset of myocardial infarction usually has a crescendo pattern). The best tests for the prompt diagnosis of aortic dissection are CT angiography and transesophageal echocardiography (transthoracic echocardiography doesn't work). When working in the emergency department, choose the one that can be done the soonest (in most hospitals, CT). Contrast aortography used to be the test of choice, but may show only one lumen (not both the true and false lumens), and thus can be misleading. Coronary angiography is not useful in diagnosis. MRI is time consuming and less cost-effective than CT angiography.

**Treatment of aortic dissection** • Treatment of dissection of the ascending aorta is immediate surgery. Intra-aortic balloon counterpulsation is contraindicated because it may cause rupture in the area of dissection. Delaying repair to allow fibrosis of the aortic wall is neither necessary nor helpful. Heparin increases the bleeding risk. For descending aortic dissections, medical management with beta blockers and afterload reduction is preferred unless a complication develops that would mandate surgery. These include rupture with bleeding, organ ischemia, uncontrolled pain, uncontrolled hypertension, and expansion of the false aneurysm.

**Complications of ascending aortic dissection** • All of the complications listed in the question may occur with dissection. Aortic valve regurgitation presents with a new murmur and decreased pulse pressure, not with distended neck veins. Dissection may occlude carotid arteries and cause stroke. Free rupture into the right chest can occur, resulting in hypovolemic shock that would present with tachycardia, decreased breath sounds on the right side, and flat neck veins. Involvement of the coronary ostia can result in myocardial infarction. However, plethora and neck vein distension are consistent with cardiac tamponade due to rupture into the pericardial sac.

**Risk factors for aortic dissection** • Hypertension and Marfan's syndrome are risk factors for aortic dissection. Atherosclerosis, while a clear risk factor in thoracic aortic aneurysm formation, is not a risk factor for dissection. Syphilis can result in aortic aneurysm formation with aneurysms that can result in aortic regurgitation and erosion into the chest wall.

**Answers** • 1-C 2-A 3-D 4-C

## CASE PRESENTATION

A 45-year-old bricklayer complains of back pain. On examination, he has weakness of left foot dorsiflexion as well as decreased sensation on his posterior left thigh, the anterior calf overlying the tibia, and onto his great toe.

1. Which of the following is the most likely cause?
   A. L4 nerve root compression from a herniated disk
   B. L5 nerve root compression from a herniated disk
   C. S1 nerve root compression from a herniated disk
   D. Muscle spasm with compression of the lumbar plexus
   E. Cauda equina syndrome
2. Which of the following is the most appropriate test to evaluate this patient's radiculopathy?
   A. Computed tomographic (CT) scan of the lumbar spine
   B. Magnetic resonance imaging (MRI) of the lumbar spine
   C. Electromyelography (EMG)
   D. Plain film of the lumbar spine
   E. Myelogram
3. A disk herniation is suspected as the cause for the patient's problems. Which of the following would be the most appropriate management at this point?
   A. Operative excision of the disk
   B. Nonsteroidal anti-inflammatory agents, muscle relaxants, and reduced activity
   C. Steroid injection into the disk space
   D. 2 weeks of bed rest with traction
   E. 2 weeks of bed rest alone
4. Which of the following would be an indication for surgery in this patient?
   A. Persistent back pain without radicular symptoms
   B. MRI showing a herniated disk between the L5 and S1 vertebrae
   C. Radicular signs and symptoms that do not respond to nonsurgical therapies
   D. All of the above
   E. None of the above

## COMMENT

**Radiculopathy** • The distribution of motor and sensory deficits in this patient is most consistent with a problem with the L5 nerve root. S1 nerve root compression would cause gastrocnemius weakness and a diminished Achilles' reflex. Compression of the L4 nerve root produces quadriceps weakness and a diminished patellar reflex. Cauda equina syndrome results from marked compression of the lumbar thecal sac and is usually manifested by bilateral deficits and sphincter dysfunction. Muscle spasm alone does not cause radiculopathy.

**Evaluation of back pain** • In the patient with radiculopathy, MRI is the most sensitive test. This study provides the best soft tissue detail and is the procedure of choice. However, where MRI is not available, or in patients in whom MRI is contraindicated, CT scan (especially CT myelogram) would be appropriate. EMG is useful only to clarify an unclear physical examination. Plain films of the spine do not show soft tissue detail and thus are unlikely to be useful in this situation. Myelography may reveal the diagnosis but is invasive and can result in complications such as spinal headache. This study also does not provide soft tissue detail. The cause of an apparent compression must be inferred based on distortions in the intrathecal dye column.

**Initial management of back pain** • Surgery is not the best initial option in the treatment of back pain and radiculopathy, even when disc herniation is confirmed on MRI or CT scan. Bed rest with or without traction is not as effective as treatment with nonsteroidal anti-inflammatory drugs, muscle relaxants, and a decrease in the patient's level of activity. Oral steroids have been tried and may provide some relief. However, these drugs are associated with a number of complications and generally are not a primary treatment method. Steroid injections into the disc space are not appropriate.

**Indications for surgery** • The presence of a disc herniation, by itself, would generally not be an indication for surgery unless the patient is symptomatic and fails to respond to conservative measures. Severe complications such as cauda equina syndrome and complete foot drop would also warrant consideration for urgent surgical therapy. In this case, the patient has symptoms related to the L5 nerve root. The L5 nerve root, like all nerve roots below the cervical spine, passes below the pedicle of the named vertebrae. Nerve root compression from disc herniation occurs at the level above the point of exit as the spinal root travels downward toward the spinal foramen. In this case, the disc between the L4 and L5 vertebra would be responsible, not the L5 S1 disc as described. Surgery to remove that disc would not improve the patient's symptoms since they do not correlate with the patient's symptoms anatomically. (This is a tricky question.)

**Answers** • 1-B 2-B 3-B 4-C

## CASE PRESENTATION

A 55-year-old man presents with 2 months of progressive bifrontal headaches and blurred vision. Physical examination is unremarkable except for papilledema.

1. Which of the following would be the best initial test?
   A. Magnetic resonance imaging (MRI) scan of the brain
   B. Noncontrasted computed tomography (CT) of the brain
   C. Lumbar puncture with cell counts and chemical analysis of fluid
   D. Angiography of the brain
   E. Electroencephalogram (EEG)
2. A lesion most compatible with tumor is identified in the parenchyma of the right frontal lobe. Which of the following is the most likely diagnosis?
   A. Meningioma
   B. Glioma
   C. Acoustic neuroma
   D. Metastatic lesion
   E. Medulloblastoma
3. An open biopsy is performed and a glioma is diagnosed. What is the most appropriate treatment at this point?
   A. Resection alone
   B. Radiation therapy to lesion with or without previous resection
   C. Chemotherapy alone
   D. No treatment
   E. Administration of steroids

## COMMENT

**Evaluation of headaches** • Headaches are a common complaint. However, persistent headaches, progressively worsening headaches, or headaches associated with neurologic symptoms (like his blurred vision) warrant attention. The presence of papilledema suggests the possibility of increased intracranial pressure. Lumbar puncture is contraindicated and is not likely to yield any useful diagnostic information. Noncontrasted CT scan of the brain is appropriate when evaluating for intracranial hemorrhage as occurs in traumatic brain injury. However, for tumor diagnosis, contrast is needed to help in identification of the lesions. MRI is the most appropriate test listed because it easily distinguishes brain lesions without the risk of contrast exposure. EEG is nonspecific and has little, if any, role in evaluation for headaches and possible brain tumors. Angiography may be done after a lesion is identified to distinguish a highly vascular tumor from primary vascular lesions such as arteriovenous malformations.

**Brain tumor types** • Of those listed, both glioma and a metastatic lesion could be present. Of these, the most likely, by far, is a metastatic lesion. Any patient with a newly diagnosed brain tumor warrants workup for malignancy in another location. Resection of a single isolated metastatic lesion to the brain may be indicated if the primary tumor is well controlled and there is no evidence of other brain metastases. Meningiomas are dural-based tumors found along the edge of the brain and are rarely seen in the parenchyma of the brain. Acoustic neuromas are tumors of the eighth cranial nerve and are located in the cerebellopontine angle, not in the frontal lobe. Medulloblastoma is a primitive cell tumor and usually occurs in the posterior fossa. It is most common in children.

**Management of glioma** • Glioma is rarely curable through surgery alone. Most advocate resection followed by radiation therapy, although some treat these lesions with radiation alone. Chemotherapy alone would not be appropriate in a resectable lesion. Chemotherapy may be useful if a previously treated tumor recurs. Steroids, alone, have no role in the primary treatment of brain tumors.

**Answers** • 1-A 2-D 3-B

## CASE PRESENTATION

A 29-year-old female patient has a blood pressure of 180/110 despite three antihypertensive medications.

1. Which of the following would suggest that this patient has essential hypertension, not curable with a surgical procedure?
   A. Age of onset between 25 and 30 years
   B. Progressive worsening of hypertension over the previous year
   C. Significant deterioration in renal function following initiation of an angiotensin-converting enzyme (ACE) inhibitor
   D. A unilateral small kidney
   E. Slow deterioration in renal function over the past 6 years
2. Which of the following is true about evaluation for surgically correctable hypertension?
   A. A decreased serum sodium level and increased serum potassium level suggest a correctable cause for hypertension.
   B. Decreased urinary 17-hydroxysteroid levels may indicate a correctable cause of hypertension.
   C. Elevated urinary vanillylmandelic acid (VMA) levels are not consistent with a surgically correctable cause of hypertension.
   D. Peripheral renin assay is the best screening test to identify renovascular causes of hypertension.
   E. Captopril renography is preferred over selective renal vein renin to screen for the presence of renovascular hypertension.
3. Angiography in this 29-year-old woman reveals a "string of beads" appearance in the left renal artery. Which of the following is likely to represent the most appropriate therapy?
   A. Long-term medical therapy with ACE inhibitors alone
   B. Percutaneous balloon angioplasty alone
   C. Iliac artery to renal artery bypass
   D. Renal endarterectomy
   E. Left nephrectomy

## COMMENT

**Signs of surgically correctable hypertension** • The most common type of hypertension is essential hypertension, and there is no surgical remedy. Surgically correctable causes of hypertension include renal artery stenosis, adrenal adenoma (producing aldosterone), pheochromocytoma (producing catecholamines), and coarctation of the aorta (upper extremity hypertension with normal leg pressure).

Hypertension with an age of onset at younger than 30 years or older than 55 years, or hypertension refractory to a three-drug regimen as well as hypertension in the presence of a bruit in the epigastrium or flank, suggests renal artery stenosis. Other signs include presence of a unilateral small kidney, sudden worsening of previously well-controlled hypertension, and sudden worsening of renal function. Worsening of renal function with initiation of ACE inhibitors also suggests a renovascular cause (creatinine rise of more than 0.3 mg/dL in 2 to 3 days).

**Laboratory screening in hypertension** • Hyperaldosteronism causes hypernatremia and hypokalemia, plus a rise in urinary 17-hydroxysteroid excretion. Pheochromocytoma causes increased urinary VMA and catecholamine levels. Coarctation of the aorta is suspected when arm exceeds leg blood pressure. Renal artery stenosis causes elevated renin, and selective renal vein sampling can identify it, but salt and water restriction as well as cessation of beta blockers and ACE inhibitors is required before this test. Captopril renography (renal scan before and 1 hour after administration of captopril) requires cessation of ACE inhibitors only, is noninvasive, and is able to detect bilateral abnormalities; this is the preferred screening test.

**Treatment of renovascular hypertension** • The most likely cause of renovascular hypertension in a young woman is fibrodysplastic disease. This is confirmed in this patient by the characteristic "string of beads" appearance typical of the medial fibrodysplastic variant of this disease. These lesions respond well to percutaneous transluminal angioplasty alone. ACE inhibitors may be contraindicated in renovascular hypertension, especially in bilateral disease, because they can cause progressive worsening of renal function. Nephrectomy is rarely indicated even with unilateral renovascular hypertension and should be considered only if the kidney is small, is producing renin, and the opposite kidney is known to have adequate function and low renin output. Bypass procedures and endarterectomy are more commonly employed in atherosclerotic renal artery stenosis (but stenting has improved results of angioplasty).

**Answers** • 1-E 2-E 3-B

## CASE PRESENTATION

A 57-year-old man with a long history of untreated heartburn undergoes esophagoscopy. Biopsies are taken just above the gastroesophageal junction and reveal columnar epithelium.

1. Which of the following is true?
   A. Antacid therapy alone is often effective in reversing this condition.
   B. Antireflux surgery is often effective at reversing this condition when antacid therapy fails.
   C. Periodic reevaluations with esophagoscopy and biopsy are indicated.
   D. Distal esophageal resection should be performed if reflux symptoms persist despite antacid therapy.
   E. All of the above are true.
2. The patient is lost to follow-up and returns 3 years later with increasing difficulty with swallowing solid foods. He is now beginning to have difficulty swallowing liquids. He has lost 45 pounds in the past 4 months. Barium swallow reveals a mass in the distal portion of the esophagus. Which of the following is true?
   A. Most esophageal malignancies are not resectable.
   B. Most esophageal tumors are benign.
   C. The most common tumor type is leiomyoma.
   D. Greater than 95% of esophageal malignancies are squamous cell carcinomas.
   E. Bronchoscopy should be performed prior to attempting resection.
3. Evaluation reveals adenocarcinoma of the esophagus adjacent to, but not invading into, the aorta. No distant metastatic lesions are identified, but the regional mediastinal lymph nodes in the region of the tumor are enlarged. Which of the following would be most appropriate in this patient?
   A. Local esophagectomy to resect the mass
   B. Esophagectomy with reconstruction
   C. Placement of feeding tubes with palliative radiation therapy to the tumor
   D. Radiation treatment alone
   E. Palliative treatment with placement of an intraesophageal tube

## COMMENT

**Barrett's esophagus** • The esophagus is normally lined with stratified squamous epithelium. Chronic acid reflux into the distal esophagus is associated with replacement of this normal epithelium with a columnar epithelium. This condition, known as Barrett's esophagus, is considered a potential precursor to development of esophageal adenocarcinoma. Unfortunately, antacid therapy may halt progression but does not usually cause reversal of the process. Periodic monitoring with esophagoscopy and biopsy is usually performed. Although Barrett's esophagus is associated with later development of cancer, this occurs in less than 20% of patients. Esophageal resection is a major procedure with considerable morbidity and is generally not performed unless high-grade dysplasia is noted in the abnormal area on biopsy. Low-grade dysplasia may be reversible, but high-grade dysplasia virtually always progresses to adenocarcinoma and generally warrants esophagectomy.

**Esophageal tumors** • Although most benign esophageal tumors are leiomyomas, less than 1% of esophageal tumors are benign. In the past, greater than 90% of tumors were squamous cell carcinomas. However, more recently there has been a trend toward a greater incidence of esophageal adenocarcinoma, with some series reporting adenocarcinoma in almost 50% of cases. Unfortunately, most esophageal cancers are not resectable at the time of diagnosis. The goal of therapy in these cases is relief of dysphagia. Long-term survival in these patients is rare. While bronchoscopy is an essential part of the evaluation of tumors of the upper and mid portions of the esophagus to rule out invasion into the trachea or bronchi, it is not necessary for tumors in the distal esophagus, which is below the level of the tracheal bifurcation. (This is a slightly tricky question, but it has been on the boards.)

**Management of esophageal tumors** • Invasion of surrounding structures and distant metastases are contraindications to esophageal resection. However, metastatic spread to local mediastinal nodes or to high lesser-curvature lymph nodes does not necessarily preclude resection. Local tumor resection is not an adequate procedure in esophageal cancer. Total esophagectomy through either a combined transabdominal and transthoracic incision or through a transhiatal approach is preferable. There is no convincing evidence that radiation provides any survival advantage either alone or as adjuvant therapy before or after resection.

**Answers** • 1-C 2-A 3-B

## CASE PRESENTATION

A 42-year-old woman undergoes a CT scan of the abdomen following a motor vehicle crash. No injuries are detected. However, in the left adrenal gland, a 3.5-cm mass is incidentally found. She has no medical problems and has had no medical complaints.

1. Which of the following is true?
   A. This is, most likely, a malignant lesion.
   B. Incisional biopsy should be performed.
   C. Fine needle aspiration of the mass should be performed.
   D. Electrolytes should be checked, and a 24-hour urine collection for urinary vanillylmandelic acid (VMA), urinary 17-ketosteroid, and 17-hydroxycorticosteroid levels should be ordered.
   E. Excisional biopsy should be performed.
2. Three months later, the patient returns complaining of headaches, palpitations, and episodes of flushing. On examination, she is hypertensive and mildly tachycardic. Which of the following is true?
   A. Urinary VMA levels are likely to be elevated.
   B. The tumor is most likely in the adrenal cortex.
   C. In some cases, this may be associated with increased serum gastrin levels.
   D. 24-hour urine output of 5-hydroxyindoleacetic acid (5-HIAA) is likely to be elevated.
   E. In some cases, Whipple's triad may be present.
3. The patient is found to have increased levels of serum epinephrine and increased catecholamine levels. No other masses are identified. The patient reports no family history of adrenal tumors or other endocrine abnormalities. Of the following, what would be the most appropriate next step in the patient's evaluation?
   A. Metaiodobenzylguanidine (MIBG) scan for localization followed by excision of the mass
   B. Alpha blockade for 1 to 3 weeks, followed by excision of the mass
   C. Beta blockade for 3 days, followed by alpha blockade for 1 to 3 weeks before excision of the mass
   D. Excision of the mass alone
   E. Beta blockade alone, followed by excision of the mass
4. After resection, which of the following should be included in the patient's management?
   A. Radiation therapy to the adrenal bed, followed by annual MIBG scan
   B. Chemotherapy, followed by annual MIBG scan
   C. Annual follow-up MIBG scans
   D. Periodic measurement of urinary VMA or catecholamine levels
   E. Both radiation therapy and chemotherapy, followed by annual MIBG scan

## COMMENT

**Evaluation of incidental adrenal mass** • Adrenal masses are present in as many as 2% of the population. While most are benign, functional (catecholamine-producing) tumors and malignancies do occur. Treatment is surgical for both. Metastatic lesions to the adrenal gland also occur. It is appropriate to assure that the incidentally found lesion is both nonfunctional and likely to be benign. Well-circumscribed, nonfunctional tumors less than 5 cm in size are rarely malignant and do not require excision unless they increase in size with time. Incisional biopsy has no place in evaluation of these lesions. Needle biopsy has no usefulness in distinguishing a benign cortical adenoma from a malignant adrenal cortical carcinoma and may induce a hypertensive crisis if the tumor proves to be a pheochromocytoma.

**Functional adrenal masses** • These symptoms in a patient with an adrenal mass are most consistent with a diagnosis of pheochromocytoma. However, only about one-third of patients have these symptoms. Nearly 50% of pheochromocytomas present as incidentally found masses. Pheochromocytomas originate in the adrenal medulla and produce catecholamines. Urinary VMA levels will be elevated in patients with pheochromocytoma. Functional cortical tumors most commonly produce aldosterone, cortisol, or sex hormones. 5-HIAA is a chemical marker of carcinoid tumor, which may present with episodic flushing as well. However, this tumor originates in the gastrointestinal tract rather than the adrenal gland. Whipple's triad consists of symptoms of hypoglycemia during fasting or exercise, serum glucose levels below 45 during these episodes, and relief of symptoms following administration of glucose. This occurs with insulinomas, which, like gastrinomas, occur largely in the region of the pancreas. Both gastrinomas and insulinomas may occur in multiple endocrine neoplasia type 1 (MEN 1). This syndrome includes pancreatic islet cell tumors, pituitary tumors, and parathyroid hyperplasia. Pheochromocytoma occurs in MEN 2A and MEN 2B.

**Management of pheochromocytoma** • Elevated urinary VMA, catecholamine, and metanephrine levels all suggest pheochromocytoma. Serum epinephrine or norepinephrine or both are also frequently elevated, but may not be in normotensive patients. MIBG scan is indicated when extra-adrenal pheochromocytoma or multiple tumor foci are suspected, such as in familial cases or in patients with MEN 2 and in patients with chemical evidence of pheochromocytoma but no apparent tumor on CT scan. CT scan alone is adequate in this case. Prior to resection, it is essential to control hypertension. Alpha-adrenergic blockade is generally started 1 to 3 weeks before surgery. These patients often are quite volume depleted. Adequate hydration must also be accomplished. If, after initiation of alpha blockade, the patient remains tachycardic, beta-adrenergic blockade should also be started. This should never be started before alpha blockade because the resultant unopposed alpha-adrenergic stimulation will worsen the patient's hypertension.

**Surgical follow-up** • Pheochromocytomas are rarely malignant. The risk is somewhat higher in female patients and in both extra-adrenal tumors and familial tumors. Unfortunately, malignant tumors often cannot be distinguished from benign lesions on pathologic examination. Even benign lesions recur in 6% to 7% of patients. Lifelong follow-up is essential. Adjuvant therapy has no role in sporadic isolated pheochromocytoma. Periodic measurement of blood pressure and urinary catecholamine metabolite levels is all that is required to screen for recurrence.

**Answers** • 1-D 2-A 3-B 4-D

# • Section 2

# Obstetrics and Gynecology

Paige R. Gernt, MD

Charles N. Landen, Jr., MD

## CASE PRESENTATION

A 37-year-old woman presents to your office and reports that during her self-exam 3 months ago she noticed a breast mass that is slightly tender and has not gone away. She has been performing self-exams for the last 15 years and has never had a mammogram or noticed a lump. Two of her mother's sisters died of breast cancer in their 60s, she has been pregnant twice, and her menses began at age 9.

1. According to the Gail model, which of the following would place a patient at increased risk of breast cancer?
   A. Prior breast biopsy
   B. Two maternal aunts with breast cancer
   C. First child delivered after age 25
   D. First period at age 15
   E. African American race
2. Of the following, which is the most accurate method of detecting early breast cancer?
   A. Breast self-exams
   B. Annual exams by a physician
   C. Mammography
   D. Ultrasound
3. On exam, which of the following would increase your suspicion of breast cancer?
   A. Size smaller than 2 cm
   B. Skin retraction
   C. Bilateral nonbloody discharge
   D. Cystic consistency
   E. Tenderness on palpation of the mass
4. Simple aspiration of the mass is unsuccessful. Fine needle aspiration is performed, and ductal carcinoma in situ is diagnosed. After excision of the mass and appropriate testing, which of the following factors best predicts the patient's prognosis?
   A. Estrogen and progesterone receptor status
   B. DNA ploidy by histogram
   C. Tumor size
   D. Patient age
   E. Presence of lymph node metastasis
5. The patient undergoes conservative breast excision with lymph node sampling. She is disease free for 7 years and presents to you reporting hot flashes, vaginal dryness, and cessation of menses. In regard to hormone replacement therapy (HRT), she should be told that:
   A. There is no randomized study examining outcomes in patients with breast cancer on HRT.
   B. As primary prevention, estrogen has been shown to decrease the incidence of cardiovascular disease (the leading cause of death in postmenopausal women) and osteoporosis.
   C. Estrogen can decrease the incidence of hot flushes, improve libido, improve vaginal dryness, and improve irritability associated with menopause.
   D. Whether or not to take HRT must be the patient's decision, taking into consideration her symptoms, the beneficial effects of HRT, and the uncertain effects on breast cancer survival.
   E. All of the above.

## COMMENT

**Gail model** • The Gail model is a method of quantifying a patient's risk of developing breast cancer. It gives both a 5-year and a lifetime risk. Factors considered in the model that increase risk include increasing patient age, earlier age of menarche, later age of first birth (after 35), increasing number of *first-degree* relatives with breast cancer, increased number of previous breast biopsies, and white race. A patient with two aunts with breast cancer may be at slightly increased risk, but the Gail model only considers affected first-degree relatives.

**Early detection** • The mammogram can, on average, detect lesions as small as 1 mm, whereas most palpable masses are at least 1 cm in diameter. On average, mammography may detect a mass 2 years before clinical examination. As a consequence of this early detection, use of mammography in women aged 50 to 70 years has been shown to reduce mortality from breast cancer by up to 30%. Ultrasound is a useful adjunct to mammography and exam, allowing distinction between cystic and solid masses. As a screening tool, however, ultrasound is not useful because its false positive and false negative rates are unacceptably high.

**Exam findings** • As breast cancer masses grow, they may become fixed to the connective tissue of the breast (Cooper's ligaments) or the underlying pectoral muscles. This may lead to dimpling of the skin or asymmetry within the breast. Mobility is decreased. The consistency of the mass is typically solid, not cystic. A unilateral bloody discharge is the most common presentation of an intraductal papilloma, and is diagnosed by excisional biopsy. Presence of any of these findings would increase the suspicion of breast cancer. Fibrocystic changes are typically tender, increase cyclically with menses, and are associated with multiple small bilateral masses.

**Prognosis in ductal carcinoma in situ** • The treatment of choice for stage I or II breast cancer is excision of the primary tumor with either lymph node dissection or sentinel lymph node biopsy, followed by radiation therapy and, in some patients, tamoxifen (if estrogen receptor testing is positive). Lymph node sampling has the best prognostic value, as the presence of positive lymph nodes decreases predicted 5-year survival by 30% to 40%. Of patients with negative nodes, however, 25% to 30% will eventually experience recurrence. Increased tumor size (greater than 2 cm) and increased DNA ploidy are associated with increased recurrence risk. Estrogen receptor status has been shown to predict a positive response to hormonal adjuvant therapy and therefore improved prognosis.

**HRT and breast cancer** • Whether to offer hormone replacement therapy to patients at high risk for, or previously diagnosed with, breast cancer is controversial. No large randomized prospective studies have been performed on HRT use in breast cancer patients, but several are in progress. More than 50 observational studies have failed to definitively show an adverse effect. Even in studies showing increased rate of breast cancer, the mortality rate is unchanged or *decreased*. Estrogen has been shown to be effective in primary prevention of cardiovascular disease and osteoporosis. Positive associations have also been seen with estrogen use and decreased incidence of colon cancer, Alzheimer's disease, and perimenopausal symptoms.

The decision to initiate HRT in any patient should be individualized. The patient's understandable fear of breast cancer should be recognized, and tempered with an explanation of the facts about cardiovascular disease and an improvement in perimenopausal symptoms.

**Answers** • 1-A 2-C 3-B 4-E 5-E

## CASE PRESENTATION

A 28-year-old woman presents to your office for her first obstetrical visit. By her last menstrual period she has an approximate 12 weeks' gestation. She has no medical problems. Her surgical history is significant for an appendectomy as a child. She is currently taking prenatal vitamins. Her obstetrical history is significant for one first trimester spontaneous abortion and one term vaginal delivery. She reports mild nausea. She denies cramping or vaginal bleeding. Her physical exam is benign except for the uterine size, palpating approximately 16 weeks. With fetal Doppler you detect two heartbeats, each approximately 150 beats per minute.

1. A pelvic ultrasound is performed. Findings of the ultrasound include two fetuses, each with a separate placenta and a thick membrane separating the fetuses. Based on this finding how would you describe the placentation?
   A. Monoamniotic, monochorionic
   B. Monoamniotic, dichorionic
   C. Diamniotic, monochorionic
   D. Diamniotic, dichorionic
   E. None of the above
2. The pregnancy nomenclature for this patient is:
   A. G4P1A1
   B. G3P1A1
   C. G4P0A1
   D. G3P2A0
   E. None of the above
3. The most common presentation of twin A followed by twin B is:
   A. Vertex/vertex
   B. Vertex/breech
   C. Breech/vertex
   D. Breech/breech
   E. All of the above are found equally
4. Serial ultrasounds for growth are ordered every 4 to 6 weeks for twin gestations. If discordant growth is noted, what must one suspect most?
   A. Rh isoimmunization
   B. Twin to twin transfusion
   C. In utero infection
   D. Gestational diabetes
   E. None of the above

## COMMENT

**Placentation** • Twin gestations are divided into two categories: dizygotic or monozygotic. Dizygotic twins result when two ova are fertilized, whereas monozygotic twins result from one ova dividing into two separate fetuses. Dizygotic twins will each have a distinct placenta with its own amnion and chorion. A *thick* membrane separating the two fetuses is often seen on ultrasound, representing the fusion of the amnions and chorions. This placentation is described as diamniotic, dichorionic. Monozygotic twins have placentation referred to as monoamniotic/monochorionic or diamniotic/monochorionic.

Monoamniotic/monochorionic indicates that one placenta is shared between the two fetuses and one amnion surrounds both fetuses. Ultrasound findings of diamniotic/monochorionic twins include one placenta shared by the two fetuses, each with a surrounding amnion. A characteristic *thin* membrane is seen separating the two fetuses. There is no placentation known as monoamniotic/dichorionic.

**Pregnancy nomenclature** • This patient's current status would be written as G3P1A1. Each separate *pregnancy* is described in the gravidity (G). Gravidity does not include the number of fetuses. She has had three pregnancies: the current pregnancy and the prior vaginal delivery and spontaneous abortion. Parity (P) indicates the number of *deliveries* greater than 20 weeks' gestation. She has only experienced one. Abortions (A) include elective terminations and miscarriages of less than 20 weeks' gestation collectively.

**Twin presentations** • The majority of twin gestation presentations are vertex/vertex, thus enabling a vaginal delivery. If the presenting twin is breech or transverse, cesarean section is recommended. Vertex/breech presents an option for the physician. A vaginal delivery of twin A followed by vaginal breech extraction of twin B may be performed; however, because newer literature suggests a poorer outcome for singleton vaginal breech deliveries, a cesarean section for delivery of both fetuses is acceptable.

**Discordant growth in twins** • Ultrasound for growth is recommended every 4 to 6 weeks after 20 weeks' gestation for all twin pregnancies. Serial growth ultrasounds will identify adequate interval growth. Lagging or no interval growth of one twin often leads to the suspicion of twin to twin transfusion syndrome. All options listed may cause growth changes, but with a twin gestation, twin to twin transfusion syndrome should be first on the differential diagnoses. This syndrome is more common in monozygotic twin gestations. The syndrome occurs when a communication exists between the arterial circulation of one twin and the venous circulation of the other twin. Because of the vascular communication, one fetus, the "donor," transfuses the "recipient." The donor fetus eventually becomes anemic and growth restricted, while the recipient becomes polycythemic and hydropic. The perinatal mortality of twin to twin transfusion syndrome may be as high as 70%.

**Answers** • 1-D 2-B 3-A 4-B

## CASE PRESENTATION

A 35-year-old G1P0 with approximately 8 weeks' gestation presents for her first obstetrical visit. After reviewing her lab results, you notice her blood type is O Rh-negative. She does not understand what this means regarding her pregnancy and wishes to discuss this further.

1. You discuss with the patient that the administration of Rh immune globulin is to protect her from becoming isoimmunized, thus affecting future pregnancies. You explain that isoimmunization occurs when:
   A. Rh-negative mother produces antibodies against red blood cells of Rh-positive fetus
   B. Rh-negative mother produces antibodies against red blood cells of Rh-negative fetus
   C. Rh-positive mother produces antibodies against red blood cells of Rh-positive fetus
   D. Rh-positive mother produces antibodies against red blood cells of Rh-negative fetus
   E. All of the above are possible etiologies of Rh isoimmunization
2. You inform her that she will be receiving the Rh immune globulin injection at both 28 weeks' gestation and after delivery. Which of the following would necessitate an additional Rh immune globulin administration during her pregnancy?
   A. Chorionic villus sampling
   B. Ectopic pregnancy
   C. External cephalic version
   D. All of the above
   E. None of the above
3. The patient conveys to you that she does not tolerate injections and would like to decline. You inform her the only situation in which Rh immune globulin would not be indicated is:
   A. If she agrees to receive Rh immune globulin with the next pregnancy
   B. If the father of the baby is Rh-negative
   C. If she decides to terminate this pregnancy
   D. If she receives Rh immune globulin at the time of her genetic amniocentesis
   E. All of the above

## COMMENT

**Etiology of isoimmunization** • Rh isoimmunization occurs in an Rh-negative mother carrying an Rh-positive fetus. Rh-negative refers to an individual whose red blood cells do not possess the D antigen. If transplacental passage of maternal and fetal blood occurs, the Rh-negative mother's body identifies Rh-positive fetal red blood cells as foreign and begins to produce antibodies against the fetal red blood cells. Antibody production leads to destruction of fetal red blood cells, resulting in severe anemia. The anemia is noted by the fetus becoming hydropic.

**Indications for Rh immune globulin administration** • Rh-negative patients routinely receive 300 $\mu g$ intramuscularly of Rh immune globulin at 28 weeks' gestation and within 72 hours of delivery. Indications for additional Rh immunoglobulin include any procedure or occurrence with a risk of transplacental passage of maternal and fetal blood. Examples include spontaneous or elective abortions, amniocenteses, chorionic villi sampling, external cephalic version, and ectopic pregnancies.

**Exception to administration of Rh immune globulin** • Of the options listed, the only acceptable reason not to administer Rh immune globulin is if the father of the fetus is Rh-negative. If the father does not wish to have his blood type drawn or if the father of the fetus is in question, Rh immune globulin should be given. Waiting until the next pregnancy is absolutely out of the question because the Rh immune globulin protects against isoimmunization that may affect the next pregnancy. Amniocentesis and termination are known indications for Rh immune globulin because of the potential risk of mixing of maternal and fetal blood.

**Answers** • 1-A 2-D 3-B

## CASE PRESENTATION

A 38-year-old G6P5 at 41 0/7 weeks has just delivered an 8 lb 2 oz male infant vaginally. A three-vessel cord placenta delivered spontaneously approximately 10 minutes after delivery. She was brought in for induction with oxytocin due to oligohydramnios. Her past medical history is significant for chronic hypertension, which has been controlled with methyldopa. Her cervical exam when arriving to labor and delivery was 1/30%/−3. She denied vaginal bleeding, leakage of fluid, or spontaneous contractions prior to labor. You notice after delivery that she begins to have brisk vaginal bleeding. Her blood pressure is 130/90 and pulse 108.

1. Which of the following is the most likely cause of this patient's bleeding?
   A. Retained products of conception
   B. Uterine atony
   C. Vaginal sidewall laceration
   D. Uterine involution
   E. None of the above
2. Which of the following would be your first line of therapy?
   A. IM ergotamine
   B. IM prostaglandin
   C. Dilatation and curettage
   D. Uterine massage
   E. None of the above
3. Which of the following would be contraindicated in this patient?
   A. IM ergotamine
   B. IM prostaglandin
   C. IV oxytocin
   D. Uterine massage
   E. All of the above
4. After all of your efforts, the bleeding continues. Which of the following should be considered?
   A. Hypogastric artery ligation
   B. Hysterectomy
   C. Uterine artery embolization
   D. All of the above
   E. None of the above

## COMMENT

**Etiology of postpartum hemorrhage** • All of the choices listed are possible causes of postpartum hemorrhage; however, atony is the most likely cause in this scenario. A multigravida who has been receiving oxytocin will often have an atonic uterus. This simply means the uterus will not contract to the appropriate size after delivery, thus continuing to bleed. Sidewall lacerations may be seen with the use of forceps or vacuum. Retained placenta is not likely because the placenta was spontaneously delivered and noted to be intact. Pieces of retained placenta may be the etiology of bleeding when manual extraction is performed. Involution of the uterus is very rare, occurring in approximately 1 in 15,000 pregnancies. Involution should be viewed as an obstetric emergency. With delivery of the placenta, the fundus of the uterus inverts, following the placenta through the cervix. The uterus must immediately be restored to its original position to prevent continued hemorrhage. Restoration may be performed vaginally using a muscle relaxant such as nitroglycerin or by laparotomy if vaginal placement is unsuccessful.

**Treatment options** • All of the choices listed are options to control postpartum hemorrhage. As atony is the most likely etiology of this patient's bleeding, the first course of action would be to provide aggressive uterine massage. Ergotamines provide vasoconstriction to decrease bleeding. Prostaglandins, such as prostaglandin $F_{2\alpha}$ (PGF2$\alpha$), produce a uterotonic effect. These two classes of drugs may be used if massage is ineffective. Because retained products are not likely, dilatation and curettage would not be warranted.

**Contraindications** • Because of the vasoconstrictive nature of ergotamines, their use is contraindicated in patients with elevated blood pressure. This includes postpartum patients with preeclampsia and chronic hypertension. Prostaglandin $F_{2\alpha}$ should not be given to known asthmatic patients due to exacerbation of symptoms. Because this patient has a known history of chronic hypertension, an ergotamine, Methergine, should not be used. Oxytocin, PGF2$\alpha$, and massage each help the uterus contract, thus correcting uterine atony.

**Continued postpartum hemorrhage** • Each answer listed is an option for correction of continued postpartum bleeding. Each method attempts to decrease the blood supply to the uterus. Uterine artery embolization is performed in the radiological suite. Angiographically directed, a polyvinyl gel is guided and placed to occlude the uterine artery. If the patient is rapidly deteriorating or if this service is unavailable, laparotomy is performed. An initial approach during laparotomy is ligation of the uterine artery or hypogastric artery. The hypogastric artery is retroperitoneal in the pelvis, and dissection may be time consuming. If excessive bleeding continues, hysterectomy may be the only choice for cessation of bleeding.

**Answers** • 1-B 2-D 3-A 4-D

## CASE PRESENTATION

A 23-year-old G0 presents to your office and reports cessation of menstrual periods over the last 7 months. She is sexually active and trying to get pregnant. She has taken multiple pregnancy tests, all of which have been negative. Her menses began at age 12 and have been regular until now. On review of systems, she has noticed an irregular milky discharge from both breasts. She is otherwise healthy. On exam, a milky, nonbloody discharge can be expressed from both breasts. There are no masses, skin retractions, or asymmetry. Pelvic exam shows a normal vagina, cervix, uterus, and adnexa.

1. Which of the following tests would be the least helpful?
   - A. Urine or serum pregnancy test
   - B. Thyroid stimulating hormone (TSH) level
   - C. Prolactin level
   - D. Magnetic resonance imaging (MRI) of the head
   - E. Progesterone challenge
2. The prolactin test returns 121 ng/mL (normal $<$40 ng/mL). The patient has a withdrawal bleed after medroxyprogesterone acetate, and upon reexamination the patient denies headaches and visual changes and does not have any focal central nervous system (CNS) findings. An MRI is ordered, which shows a microadenoma in the anterior pituitary. What is the best therapy for this patient?
   - A. Observation with frequent prolactin checks
   - B. Initiation of oral contraceptives
   - C. Initiation of bromocriptine (Parlodel)
   - D. Ovulation induction with clomiphene citrate
   - E. Radiation therapy
3. Which of the following conditions may be associated with galactorrhea?
   - A. Graves' disease
   - B. Antipsychotic medication
   - C. Use of low dose oral contraceptives
   - D. Ductal carcinoma
   - E. Fibrocystic breast disease

**Answers** • 1-D 2-C 3-B

## COMMENT

**Evaluation of galactorrhea** • The patient's current diagnosis is secondary amenorrhea. The most common cause of this is pregnancy, and a pregnancy test should be obtained, despite her repeatedly negative tests. Any patient with secondary amenorrhea and a negative pregnancy test should have TSH and prolactin levels checked. Hypothyroidism, hyperthyroidism, and high prolactin can interfere with the pulsatile release in gonadotropin releasing hormone (GnRH), preventing follicle-stimulating hormone (FSH) and luteinizing hormone (LH) release. The progesterone challenge is a clinical test that determines whether estrogen is being produced in sufficient quantities to allow proliferation of the endometrium. If estrogen is present in sufficient quantities, the patient will have menses a couple of days after the progesterone course ends. This suggests an anovulation problem. An MRI of the head is indicated only if the prolactin is significantly elevated. If a workup is negative, an FSH level can be measured to evaluate for premature ovarian failure.

**Management of prolactin microadenoma** • The management options for a pituitary microadenoma are broad and depend primarily on the patient's discomfort with symptoms. Microadenomas infrequently grow to a size at which they cause other pituitary problems. They are rarely invasive, especially when prolactin levels are less than 1000 ng/mL; therefore, microadenomas are rarely dangerous in and of themselves. In a patient who is not bothered by absence of menses or galactorrhea, observation with routine prolactin level checks is appropriate. Treatment centers on management of two primary clinical symptoms: anovulation and galactorrhea.

Bromocriptine (Parlodel) and cabergoline (Dostinex) are dopamine agonists that decrease prolactin levels and will usually suppress a microadenoma to where it is undetectable. Most patients will resume menses, and if fertility is desired, be able to conceive. Dopamine agonist therapy is even effective in 90% of cases for large *macroadenomas*. It is the recommended treatment for prolactinomas. Oral contraceptive therapy corrects amenorrhea caused by hyperprolactinemia and is an excellent way to replace estrogen in estrogen-deficient women. Unlike dopamine agonists, oral contraceptives will not reduce microadenomas. Radiation therapy and surgery are not indicated for primary management of microadenomas. Even with macroadenomas (more than 1 cm on MRI), radiation and surgery are only curative in about 50% of cases.

Because this patient is trying to get pregnant, starting a dopamine agonist is the best management. Ovulation induction is appropriate for women with unexplained anovulation, but in this case, correction of the underlying problem is likely to allow ovulation.

**Causes of galactorrhea** • Galactorrhea results from a hormonal imbalance of prolactin or estrogen or both. A ductal carcinoma typically presents as a unilateral bloody nipple discharge. Bilateral galactorrhea would point to a hormonal problem. Prolactin excess is most commonly caused by a prolactinoma. Prolactin secretion is *inhibited* by prolactin-inhibiting factor (PIF), which is probably dopamine. Therefore, dopamine antagonists such as antipsychotics can lead to hyperprolactinemia. Prolactin secretion is *stimulated* by thyroid-releasing factor (TRH). Increased TRH and galactorrhea usually result from hypothyroidism. Treatment of these conditions is correction of the underlying problem or use of a dopamine agonist. In Graves' disease, TRH is low because of excess thyroid hormone production. Cases of estrogen excess causing galactorrhea include early pregnancy, the postpartum period, high-dose oral contraceptives, and obesity. Treatment is correction of the underlying problem, reassurance, or change to low-dose oral contraceptives.

## ● CASE PRESENTATION

A 29-year-old African American G2P1 at 28 1/7 weeks is seen in your office for her routine obstetrical visit. She has no complaints. She denies loss of fluid, vaginal bleeding, or contractions. She reports good fetal movement. Her obstetrical history is significant for spontaneous vaginal delivery of an infant weighing 4600 g. Her past medical history is negative. Her family history is significant for hypertension and diabetes mellitus. She does not smoke or drink alcohol. Overall, her pregnancy has been uneventful. Her 1-hour glucose tolerance test is performed and returns 153 mg/dL.

1. Which of the following in her history is an indication for the 1-hour glucose tolerance test?
   A. African American ethnicity
   B. 29 years of age
   C. Positive family history
   D. Previous infant weighing more than 4500 g
   E. All of the above
2. Because the 1-hour glucose test result is greater than 140, you decide to perform a 3-hour, 100 g, glucose tolerance test. Which of the following indicates the patient has the diagnosis of gestational diabetes?

| | Fasting | 1 hour | 2 hours | 3 hours |
|---|---|---|---|---|
| A. | 95 | 180 | 150 | 135 |
| B. | 110 | 194 | 168 | 135 |
| C. | 103 | 173 | 144 | 120 |
| D. | 98 | 186 | 135 | 123 |
| E. | 90 | 165 | 140 | 140 |

3. Which of the following would be your next course of action?
   A. Begin subcutaneous insulin injections
   B. Place on oral hypoglycemic
   C. Begin IV insulin
   D. Place on American Diabetic Association diet
   E. No action needed because this patient does not have gestational diabetes
4. Which of the following is *not* a risk factor associated with gestational diabetes?
   A. Risk of continued insulin resistance
   B. Risk of intrauterine growth restriction
   C. Risk of macrosomia
   D. Risk of shoulder dystocia
   E. None of the above
5. During delivery of the infant a shoulder dystocia is encountered. Which of the following maneuvers is contraindicated?
   A. McRoberts' position
   B. Suprapubic pressure
   C. Delivery of the posterior arm
   D. Fundal pressure

## ● COMMENT

**Screening for gestational diabetes** • Many practices no longer institute universal gestational diabetes screening. A 1-hour 50 g glucose tolerance test is administered to patients with risk factors for gestational diabetes. African American and Hispanic ethnicities have an increased incidence of gestational diabetes compared to Caucasians. Other risk factors include a history of gestational diabetes with a previous pregnancy, delivery of an infant weighing more than 4500 g, family history of diabetes mellitus, and patients older than 25 years.

**Three-hour glucose tolerance test** • If the 1-hour 50 g glucose tolerance test result is greater than 140 mg/dL, a 3-hour 100 g glucose tolerance test should be performed. If any two values of the 3-hour glucose tolerance test are abnormal, the diagnosis of gestational diabetes is given. Values include a serum fasting, 1-hour, 2-hour, and 3-hour level. The normal values of these are as follows: fasting, less than 105 mg/dL; 1 hour, less than 190 mg/dL; 2 hour, less than 165 mg/dL; 3 hour, less than 145 mg/dL.

**Treatment of gestational diabetes** • Because this patient does have the diagnosis of gestational diabetes, the first course of action would be to begin an 1800- to 2200-Kcal per day American Diabetic Association diet. The patient should be instructed by a nutritionist and taught performance of finger stick glucose levels. If by diet alone the patient keeps her fasting glucose levels less than 105 mg/dL and her 2-hour postprandial levels less than 120 mg/dL, no further intervention is necessary. If this is not obtained by diet alone, the next step is insulin therapy.

**Risk factors** • Patients with poorly controlled gestational diabetes have an increased risk of macrosomia. Macrosomia results as increased maternal glucose crosses the placenta, causing fetal hyperglycemia and fetal hyperinsulinemia. Fetal insulin possesses a growth hormone-like effect, leading to excessive adipose deposition and fetal growth. Macrosomia increases the risk of shoulder dystocia. Patients with gestational diabetes who require insulin should be screened at their 6 weeks' postpartum visit for continued insulin resistance. Fetuses of patients with gestational diabetes do not appear to be at an increased risk for intrauterine growth restriction. Growth restriction may be seen in patients with type 1 or type 2 diabetes mellitus.

**Shoulder dystocia** • When a shoulder dystocia is encountered, several maneuvers are advocated. The patient should be placed in McRoberts' position. This position includes flexion of the hips to widen the pelvic outlet. Suprapubic pressure is applied to help the anterior shoulder move under the pubic symphysis. Fundal pressure should *not* be applied, because this does not aid in relieving the anterior shoulder and may cause fetal trauma. If other maneuvers are not helpful, the posterior arm may be delivered, causing collapse of the anterior shoulder and successful delivery.

**Answers** • 1-E 2-B 3-C 4-B 5-D

## CASE PRESENTATION

A 25-year-old woman presents to your office after palpating a small mass upon self-breast examination. She states this has never been present before and is quite concerned. A paternal aunt was diagnosed with infiltrating ductal carcinoma three years ago. She reports occasional tenderness of bilateral breasts, with tenderness worse at time of menses. She denies nipple discharge. She denies recent trauma to the chest or breasts. Upon physical examination, the breasts are symmetrical without dimpling or skin changes. No lymphadenopathy is identified. A 1 cm by 1 cm slightly tender, mobile, well-circumscribed mass is palpated in the right upper outer quadrant. The left breast is without significant findings.

1. After performing the history and physical, the most likely diagnosis is:
   A. Fibrocyst
   B. Fibroadenoma
   C. Infiltrating ductal carcinoma
   D. Fat necrosis
   E. None of the above
2. You decide to proceed with needle aspiration of the mass. You would expect to see:
   A. Blood
   B. Nothing retrieved with aspiration
   C. Straw-colored fluid
   D. All of the above
   E. None of the above
3. After aspiration you would expect this mass to be:
   A. Approximately the same size
   B. Collapsed/resolved
   C. Half of its original size
   D. Doubled in size
   E. None of the above
4. The next step in the management of this patient is:
   A. Referral to a breast surgeon
   B. Mammogram
   C. Clinical breast exam in 1 to 2 months
   D. All of the above
   E. None of the above

## COMMENT

**History and physical findings associated with a fibrocyst** • The most likely diagnosis is fibrocyst. A well-circumscribed, mobile, tender mass at time of menses is consistent with a fibrocyst. Fibrocysts or fibrocystic changes of the breast are usually found in reproductive-aged women, commonly ages 20 to 50. The etiology is thought to be an exaggerated response of breast tissue to cyclic hormonal changes. Breast discharge may be seen in individuals with fibrocysts. History may reveal increased caffeine consumption, but this is disputed by some authorities. The diagnosis of fibrocysts should be regarded as benign. Fibroadenomas are nontender, rubbery, solid, benign masses. Fibroadenomas are characteristically found in adolescents and women in their 20s, but may be found at any age. Growth of fibroadenomas can be rapid. Rapid growth usually leads to palpation and resultant biopsy. Invasive carcinoma is a possibility but would be unusual in someone of this age group. Characteristics associated with breast cancer include nipple inversion, skin changes known as *peau d'orange*, lymphadenopathy, and bloody nipple discharge. A malignant mass is often irregular in borders and adherent to the chest wall. Fat necrosis would be unlikely, because this is a result of trauma to the breast. Fat necrosis may present as a tender, irregular mass with skin retraction. Because of the similar characteristics of fat necrosis and carcinoma, excisional biopsy is warranted.

**Needle aspiration** • Diagnosis of a fibrocyst can be made by simple needle aspiration. The typical finding of a fibrocyst aspiration is straw-colored fluid. If no fluid is retrieved a solid mass is assumed. Because a solid mass may be a fibroadenoma or a more worrisome finding such as carcinoma, additional testing with core biopsy or excisional biopsy is needed. Aspiration of blood from a breast mass is suggestive of carcinoma. Biopsy is needed if carcinoma is suspected. This is typically performed by a surgical oncologist.

**Resolution of a breast mass** • Aspiration of a breast mass can be diagnostic. If a breast mass with straw-colored fluid resolves or disappears after aspiration, the diagnosis of fibrocyst may be made. One would not expect the size to increase or stay the same. If the mass does not completely resolve, another diagnostic test is ordered. Ultrasound of the breast is helpful because it reveals if a structure is cystic or solid.

**Additional testing** • If straw-colored fluid is retrieved upon aspiration as well as resolution of cyst, one can feel confident with the diagnosis of fibrocyst. No further diagnostic tests such as mammogram or excisional biopsy are warranted. The patient should continue self-examination of breasts and be made aware that fibrocysts often recur. A clinical exam by a physician should be repeated after one or two menstrual cycles. If no fluid is retrieved and there is the suspicion of a solid mass, other options are available. Ultrasound of the breast may be performed to identify a cystic or solid mass. If a cystic mass is visualized, needle aspiration under ultrasound guidance is performed. If the mass is solid in appearance, the decision may be to proceed with mammography or a biopsy for pathological diagnosis.

**Answers** • 1-A 2-C 3-B 4-C

## CASE PRESENTATION

A man, aged 32, and his wife, aged 28, come to your office to discuss their inability to conceive. They have been actively trying to conceive for approximately 18 months with no success. When taking the woman's history, she reports menarche at age 13 and menses every 28 days lasting 5 days. She states she has had no surgeries and has no significant past medical history. Her gynecologic history is significant for a history of pelvic inflammatory disease approximately 4 years ago. She is currently taking no medications. Husband reports no significant past medical history or surgical history. He denies having mumps. He does not take any medications or use recreational drugs. He is a lawyer. He has one child from a previous marriage.

1. The correct definition of *infertility* is:
   A. Inability to conceive after 6 months of unprotected coitus
   B. Inability to conceive after 12 months of unprotected coitus
   C. Inability to conceive after 18 months of unprotected coitus
   D. Inability to conceive after 24 months of unprotected coitus
   E. None of the above
2. Infertility may be attributed to the following causes:
   A. Male factor: semen abnormality
   B. Female factor: ovulatory dysfunction
   C. Female factor: tubal pathology
   D. All of the above
   E. None of the above
3. Which of the following is the most likely reason for this couple's inability to conceive?
   A. Decreased sperm count
   B. Undiagnosed autoimmune disease
   C. Previous pelvic inflammatory disease
   D. Anovulation
   E. None of the above
4. Which of the following tests would most likely help prove this etiology?
   A. Serum thyroid-stimulating hormone (TSH) level
   B. Semen analysis
   C. Basal body temperature chart
   D. Hysterosalpingogram
   E. None of the above
5. Your test does confirm your suspicion. Which of the following will increase the couple's chances of pregnancy?
   A. Intrauterine insemination
   B. Oral clomiphene citrate
   C. Oral doxycycline
   D. In vitro fertilization
   E. All of the above

## COMMENT

**Definition of infertility** • Infertility is defined as the inability to conceive after 1 year of unprotected coitus. Infertility affects approximately 15% of reproductive-aged couples. Approximately 50% of couples who have not conceived within 1 year will achieve a successful spontaneous pregnancy without intervention within the following year.

**Etiologies of infertility** • Infertility etiologies can be broken down into three large categories. Male factor includes problems with semen sperm count, motility, or morphology. Female factor can be divided into two categories: 1) ovulatory and 2) structural. These include decreased ovulation (e.g., polycystic ovarian disease) or decreased number of ova (e.g., premature ovarian failure). Structural reasons include distorted fallopian tubes due to scarring from a previous inflammatory reaction and distorted uterine cavity due to fibroid tumors or Müllerian anomaly.

**Tubal pathology** • Because this patient has had a prior episode of pelvic inflammatory disease, a tubal etiology should be first on the list of differential diagnoses. Her ovulatory function is most likely satisfactory since she has normal, monthly menses. Her husband has fathered one child during a previous relationship, which decreases the suspicion of male factor etiology. He has no environmental or occupational factors that lead to semen changes, such as radiation, heat, or marijuana exposure.

**Diagnostic tests** • If a structural defect is suspected, the most helpful test is a hysterosalpingogram. A radiopaque solution is injected into the cervical canal. Using fluoroscopy, the architecture of the uterine cavity and patency of the fallopian tubes can be visualized. Ovulatory dysfunction, often manifested as amenorrhea, is found by taking a menstrual history. A serum TSH and prolactin level may be beneficial, because hyperprolactinemia and hypothyroidism are both known causes of amenorrhea. Increased levels of thyrotropin-releasing hormone found in hypothyroid patients appear to stimulate prolactin-secreting cells, thus leading to hyperprolactinemia and anovulation. Basal body temperature charting is the least expensive method to detect ovulation. The patient records her temperature each morning upon rising. Ovulation is followed by an increase in body temperature. The increase in body temperature may be as small as 0.5° Fahrenheit. Because of the small change in temperature, recording may be difficult to interpret.

**Treatment options** • With distortion of the fallopian tubes, the ova and sperm are unable to unite for fertilization to occur. In vitro fertilization would be the only option for this couple. Clomiphene citrate, an antiestrogen, causes release of follicle-stimulating hormone, which in turn causes ovulation. Clomiphene citrate is the treatment of choice for ovulatory dysfunction as seen in patients with polycystic ovarian syndrome. Doxycycline and cephalosporins are used to treat pelvic inflammatory disease but would not be helpful now regarding infertility. Intrauterine insemination would not be useful, as the ovum is still unable to travel through the fallopian tube for fertilization.

**Answers** • 1-B 2-D 3-C 4-D 5-D

## CASE PRESENTATION

An 18-year-old G1P1 with no known allergies presents to your office complaining of diffuse lower abdominal pain for the last 2 days. She reports subjective fever and chills. She denies nausea, vomiting, or dysuria. She reports yellow vaginal discharge. She is sexually active and uses oral contraceptive pills for birth control. She has had two male partners in the last year. Physical examination reveals temperature 100.8°F, abdomen soft, positive guarding, no rebound, diffuse tenderness to palpation, no distension. Pelvic exam reveals vagina with yellow discharge at os, cervix erythematous, uterus small, normal size. Tenderness is noted with cervical movement and palpation over uterus and bilateral adnexa. No masses are appreciated. Urine human chorionic gonadotropin (hCG) is negative. White blood cell count is 17,000.

1. A wet prep is performed. Which of the following do you most likely expect to see upon microscopic exam?
   A. Hyphae
   B. Sheets of red blood cells
   C. Clue cells
   D. Sheets of white blood cells
   E. None of the above
2. After performing history and physical and reviewing lab results, your working diagnosis is:
   A. Appendicitis
   B. Vaginal candidiasis
   C. Ectopic pregnancy
   D. Pelvic inflammatory disease
   E. None of the above
3. The etiology of the patient's diagnosis is:
   A. *Neisseria gonorrhoeae*
   B. *Chlamydia trachomatis*
   C. *Mycoplasma hominis*
   D. *Bacteroides fragilis*
   E. All of the above
4. Of the following choices, which would be the best option for treatment according to Centers for Disease Control guidelines?
   A. IV metronidazole and IV vancomycin
   B. PO metronidazole and PO erythromycin
   C. IV ceftriaxone and IV doxycycline
   D. IM ceftriaxone and PO doxycycline
   E. None of the above
5. Which of the following would be possible sequelae of her diagnosis?
   A. Infertility
   B. Ectopic pregnancy
   C. Adhesive disease/pelvic pain
   D. All of the above
   E. None of the above

## COMMENT

**Wet prep findings** • This patient's history and physical are consistent with pelvic inflammatory disease (PID). Evaluation of vaginal discharge by wet prep in a patient with PID would reveal sheets of white blood cells, commonly referred to as *leukorrhea*. Hyphae or pseudohyphae are indicative of *Candida* species. Occasional red blood cells may be seen with inflammation of the cervix; however, one would not expect sheets of red blood cells unless active bleeding were present. Clue cells are characteristic of bacterial vaginosis. Clue cells represent vaginal epithelial cells with clusters of adherent bacteria.

**Signs and symptoms** • With abdominal pain, fever, vaginal discharge, and leukorrhea in a sexually active woman, the most likely diagnosis is pelvic inflammatory disease. Although appendicitis symptomatology is often similar, taking a thorough sexual history and performing a pelvic exam will often help differentiate the diagnoses. It is not uncommon for laparoscopy to be performed for presumed appendicitis and salpingitis with pus-like material to be found. Ectopic pregnancy may present with abdominal pain but is not typically accompanied by fever and vaginal discharge. Unstable vital signs due to intra-abdominal bleeding would suggest an ectopic pregnancy. A βhCG can be drawn to eliminate this diagnosis. Fever or uterine tenderness does not accompany vulvovaginal candidiasis. Patients complain of white, thick, cottage cheese–like vaginal discharge with itching.

**Etiology of pelvic inflammatory disease** • PID is the ascension of a polymicrobial infection from the lower genital tract to the endometrium and adnexa. All answers listed are possibilities. Cultures taken from patients with PID have revealed several aerobic, anaerobic, and atypical organisms. The most common organisms found include *Neisseria gonorrhoeae* and *Chlamydia trachomatis*. These organisms coexist in approximately 50% of cases.

**Treatment options** • The Centers for Disease Control guidelines for ambulatory or outpatient management of PID include the following: (1) Cefoxitin 2 g intramuscularly plus probenecid 1 g orally, or ceftriaxone 250 g intramuscularly plus doxycycline 100 mg orally twice a day for 14 days; (2) ofloxacin 400 mg orally twice a day for 14 days plus either clindamycin 450 mg orally four times a day or metronidazole 500 mg orally twice a day for 14 days. This patient may be treated on an outpatient basis; therefore, IM ceftriaxone and a 14-day course of doxycycline would be the optimal choice. Inpatient treatment is warranted for patients unable to tolerate oral medications due to nausea and vomiting, immunosuppressed patients, evidence of tubo-ovarian abscess, pregnancy, and if the diagnosis is uncertain. Inpatient therapy consists of (1) cefoxitin 2 g IV every 6 hours plus 100 mg doxycycline orally or IV; (2) clindamycin 900 mg IV every 8 hours plus gentamicin 2 mg/kg loading dose followed by 1.5 mg/kg maintenance dose every 8 hours.

**Sequelae of pelvic inflammatory disease** • All of the choices listed may be complications associated with pelvic inflammatory disease. With one episode of PID, fertility is decreased by approximately 12%; two episodes, 25%; and by the third episode, 50%. Ectopic pregnancy due to tubal distortion also increases with each episode of pelvic inflammatory disease. Due to scarring and adhesion formation, many patients will present with abdominal and pelvic pain that is difficult to alleviate.

**Answers** • 1-D 2-D 3-E 4-D 5-D

## CASE PRESENTATION

A 22-year-old G1P1 presents to your office complaining of a 2-day history of sporadic sharp pain in the left lower quadrant increasing in severity. She reports no vaginal discharge but occasional vaginal spotting. Her menstrual history is significant for periods every 28 days 5 days in length. She is sexually active. She has a history of *Chlamydia trachomatis* that was treated last year. She denies fever, chills, nausea, or vomiting. She denies anorexia and has noticed no change in bowel or bladder habits. On physical exam her temperature is 98.7°F, blood pressure 126/68, pulse 88 beats per minute, and respirations 20. Abdomen is soft, tender to palpation in the left lower quadrant, positive guarding, no rebound. Pelvic examination reveals a small amount of blood in vagina, cervix without discharge, os closed. Uterus is normal size, nontender, anteverted, and mobile. Palpation of a tender, 3 cm by 4 cm mass is noted in the left adnexa. Lab tests return with white blood count 7000, hemoglobin 11, and beta human chorionic gonadotropin (βhCG ) 4500 mIU/mL. She reports that a βhCG performed 2 days ago was 3900 mIU/mL.

1. The most appropriate next step in this patient's management would be:
   A. Order pelvic ultrasound
   B. Follow-up at physician's office in 1 week for new obstetric visit
   C. Order abdominal CT
   D. Schedule patient for dilatation and curettage
   E. None of the above
2. Your management revealed no evidence of an intrauterine pregnancy. The most likely diagnosis is:
   A. Complete abortion
   B. Molar pregnancy
   C. Ectopic pregnancy
   D. Incomplete abortion
   E. None of the above
3. If a normal intrauterine pregnancy had been noted, the βhCG value of 4500 mIU/mL should have been approximately:
   A. 3500
   B. 4000
   C. 5000
   D. 7500
   E. 9000
4. Which of the following is not an option for further management of this patient?
   A. Chemotherapy
   B. Discharge patient home with follow-up in 2 weeks
   C. Laparotomy
   D. Laparoscopy
   E. None of the above
5. Which of the following conditions would be an absolute contraindication for *medical* management of this patient?
   A. βhCG greater than 5000 mIU/mL
   B. Evidence of ectopic pregnancy in adnexa by ultrasound
   C. Blood pressure of 80/40 and pulse of 130 beats per minute
   D. All of the above
   E. None of the above

## COMMENT

**Diagnostic tests** • With a positive βhCG and abdominal pain, the most appropriate management is to confirm an intrauterine pregnancy. With a βhCG of approximately 6000 mIU/mL, abdominal ultrasound can confirm an intrauterine pregnancy. However, many women with ectopic pregnancies present with a βhCG value much lower than 6000 mIU/mL. With the development of the transvaginal approach, a gestational sac can be visualized with a βhCG of 2000 mIU/mL. This patient has a βhCG of 4500 mIU/mL. If no intrauterine pregnancy is seen, ectopic pregnancy is assumed and the patient should not be discharged home for follow-up. A CT scan would be beneficial to rule out other etiologies of abdominal pain, but would not be indicated as the first line of treatment. Dilatation and curettage would be indicated for treatment of an incomplete abortion. An incomplete abortion would be suspected with continued bleeding and a falling βhCG.

**Ultrasound findings** • The most likely diagnosis is an ectopic pregnancy. This is characterized by an abnormally rising βhCG, no intrauterine pregnancy visualized by ultrasound, and abdominal pain. A molar pregnancy is characterized by vaginal bleeding and an extremely elevated βhCG. βhCG levels for a molar pregnancy are often greater than 100,000 mIU/mL. Other findings associated with molar pregnancies include increased blood pressure, nausea, and the characteristic "snowstorm" appearance on ultrasound representing hydropic villi. Ultrasound findings and physical exam help make the diagnosis of complete versus incomplete abortion. Complete abortions typically have a low βhCG because products of conception have been expelled. The patient will usually give a history of abdominal cramping and passage of large clots or "tissue." Physical exam reveals minimal bleeding, closed cervical os, and no evidence of intrauterine pregnancy by ultrasound. An incomplete abortion typically is characterized by vaginal bleeding, an open os, and evidence of products of conception.

**βhCG abnormalities** • The βhCG of a normal intrauterine pregnancy prior to 10 weeks should approximately double within 48 hours. Most pregnancies experience a 66% to 100% rise in 48 hours; thus, the correct answer would be approximately 7500. The βhCG level will peak at 10 weeks and then decline throughout the rest of the pregnancy.

**Treatment options** • With the diagnosis of ectopic pregnancy in a stable patient there are different treatment options to be considered. Methotrexate 50 mg/m$^2$ IM can be administered, with a repeat βhCG drawn day 4 and day 7 postinjection. If a 15% decline in the βhCG level between day 4 and day 7 is noted, the patient is responding to treatment and weekly βhCG should be drawn and followed to zero. If a 15% decline has not been noted, a second injection of methotrexate 50 mg/m$^2$ IM should be administered. Surgery via laparotomy or laparoscopy is indicated for the patient who is not clinically stable or declines methotrexate therapy. The recovery from laparoscopy is often shorter in duration.

**Contraindications to methotrexate therapy** • There are several *relative* contraindications to methotrexate therapy. These include βhCG greater than15,000, evidence of cardiac activity of ectopic, and ectopic diameter greater than 3.5 cm. The only absolute contraindication to medical therapy is evidence of an unstable patient. This patient is tachycardiac and hypotensive. She would not be a candidate for methotrexate therapy and should proceed immediately to surgery.

**Answers** • 1-A 2-C 3-D 4-B 5-C

## CASE PRESENTATION

A 20-year-old G3P0A2 with last normal menstrual period 6 weeks ago presents to your clinic complaining of 3 days of vaginal spotting. She has been attempting pregnancy for 4 months, and had a positive pregnancy test 1 week ago. She has had no cramping or abdominal pain. She has had two prior miscarriages in the first trimester, one requiring dilation and curettage. She is otherwise healthy. On physical exam her abdomen is nontender. The vagina has a small amount of old blood in the vault, and the cervix is closed. The uterus is 6 to 8 weeks' size and nontender. A urine pregnancy test is positive.

1. The initial diagnosis is:
   A. Ectopic pregnancy
   B. Threatened abortion
   C. Incomplete abortion
   D. Complete abortion
   E. Missed abortion
2. Which of the following is not useful at this time?
   A. βhCG
   B. Transvaginal ultrasound
   C. Complete blood count (CBC)
   D. Blood type and screen
   E. Two units of cross-matched blood
3. An ultrasound shows an endometrial stripe of 10 mm with no intrauterine pregnancy visible. The adnexa are normal, with a 2-cm simple cyst, and no evidence of ectopic pregnancy. The βhCG is 1250 mIU/mL. The most appropriate next step is:
   A. Give precautions on bleeding or pain, and repeat visit in 1 week
   B. Tell the patient a miscarriage is occurring and she should allow it to pass naturally
   C. Tell the patient a miscarriage is occurring and a dilation and curettage is necessary
   D. Give precautions on bleeding or pain, and repeat βhCG in 48 hours
   E. Diagnostic laparoscopy to evaluate for ectopic pregnancy
4. The patient goes on to have a complete miscarriage. In regard to the patient's recurrent miscarriages, she should be told that:
   A. A workup is indicated if she wishes.
   B. Her risk of another miscarriage is 75%.
   C. She should have been evaluated for a cause after her first miscarriage.
   D. This pregnancy probably failed because of an underlying maternal medical condition.
   E. This pregnancy probably failed because of a maternal or paternal chromosomal abnormality.

**Answers:** • 1-B 2-E 3-D 4-A

## COMMENT

**Threatened abortion** • *Threatened abortion* is the term applied to a pregnancy with vaginal bleeding if a more specific diagnosis cannot be made with certainty. About 25% of normal pregnancies have vaginal bleeding in the first trimester.

An ectopic pregnancy, or pregnancy outside of the intrauterine cavity, cannot be confirmed with the information given. An incomplete abortion is diagnosed when products of conception are passed but tissue is still present in the intrauterine cavity. A completed abortion is diagnosed when passage of products of conception is confirmed and no tissue remains in the uterus. When a miscarriage occurs without symptoms (being discovered by incidental ultrasound), the diagnosis of missed abortion is made.

**Laboratory analysis** • Any pregnant patient with abdominal pain or vaginal bleeding should have a βhCG and ultrasound to evaluate for an ectopic pregnancy. Any pregnant patient with vaginal bleeding should have a blood type and screen, so that if the patient is Rh-negative, Rh immune globulin can be administered for prevention of isoimmunization. Even if minimal blood loss has occurred, a CBC gives a baseline in case more significant blood loss occurs. Ordering cross-matched blood at this time is premature, but would be appropriate if the patient became unstable.

**Management of miscarriage** • As often occurs with a very early pregnancy and symptoms of bleeding or pain, the specific diagnosis is not clear (a threatened abortion by definition). The differential diagnosis includes a normal pregnancy, a miscarriage at any stage (from early to completed), and an ectopic pregnancy. A dilation and curettage should not be performed if the pregnancy is desired. A diagnostic laparoscopy is indicated only if an ectopic pregnancy is diagnosed and surgical correction is desired, or if the patient is unstable and a diagnosis must be made.

When the diagnosis is unclear, βhCG levels should be followed. If the βhCG does not increase by at least 66% in a 48-hour period, an abnormal pregnancy, either miscarriage or ectopic, is strongly suggested. If the βhCG reaches 2000 mIU/mL and an intrauterine gestation is not seen by transvaginal ultrasound (or βhCG 6000 is mIU/mL for transabdominal ultrasound), an ectopic pregnancy should be strongly suspected. In these cases, an endometrial curettage can be performed in an attempt to identify villous tissue. If products of conception are identified on pathologic specimen, an ectopic pregnancy is virtually excluded. The incidence of heterotopic pregnancy, in which there is a concurrent intrauterine and ectopic pregnancy, is about 1:10,000.

**Recurrent abortions** • It is estimated that 40% to 50% of pregnancies result in miscarriage, though most go unrecognized. Approximately 15% to 20% of clinically recognized pregnancies end in miscarriage. A workup after a single miscarriage is unnecessary, costly, and increases patient anxiety. A workup is usually recommended after three consecutive miscarriages have occurred.

Based on statistical calculations, it was once thought that after three consecutive spontaneous abortions, the risk of another abortion was 75% to 80%. It is now known that this risk is only about 40%. A workup for recurrent abortions includes chromosomal analysis of the parents (a positive finding in only 2% to 4% of cases), thyroid-stimulating hormone (TSH) level, anticardiolipin antibody, lupus anticoagulant, factor V Leiden, diabetes screen, and either hysterosalpingogram or transvaginal ultrasound with saline infusion to evaluate for intrauterine structural abnormalities. Selective testing to limit costs is appropriate if a patient's clinical history suggests a more likely cause.

## CASE PRESENTATION

A 20-year-old white woman presents for an annual exam. She is using condoms for birth control, has been sexually active with one partner for 2 years, and has never had a pelvic exam. She has been in good health, but currently smokes a pack of cigarettes a day. Because she is embarrassed, she wants to know if she absolutely needs a pelvic exam with a Pap smear. She has no gynecologic complaints, including no irregular menses, discharge, or odor.

1. Which of the following is an independent risk factor for developing cervical dysplasia?
   - A. Intercourse with a single partner
   - B. Starting intercourse late in life
   - C. Infection with human papilloma virus (HPV)
   - D. Cocaine abuse
   - E. Infection with syphilis
2. Which of the following is a characteristic of a screening test?
   - A. It can identify precursor lesions with a high degree of specificity.
   - B. Treatment of the disease being screened reduces incidence of long-term sequelae.
   - C. The test is only available to select populations.
   - D. It can make a specific diagnosis and allow treatment based on the result.
   - E. The disease being screened is uncommon with a high mortality rate.
3. Pap smears are recommended:
   - A. When a woman becomes sexually active
   - B. Starting at age 18 if not yet sexually active
   - C. Yearly in the presence of risk factors
   - D. Every 1 to 3 years if she has had three consecutive negative Pap smears and no new risk factors such as new partners or having a sexually transmitted disease, and is HIV negative
   - E. All of the above
4. Which of the following is true about screening for cervical cancer?
   - A. The high-risk area of the cervix is the upper endocervical canal.
   - B. Patients with HPV types 16, 18, and 31 are at decreased risk of cervical cancer.
   - C. DNA typing of HPV subtypes should be performed with all routine cervical cancer screening.
   - D. An "unsatisfactory" Pap smear means that atypical squamous cells are noted.
   - E. Annual Pap smear testing reduces cervical cancer mortality by 90%.

## COMMENT

**Risk factors for cervical dysplasia** • There is a strong association between infection with human papilloma virus and cervical neoplasia. Epidemiologically, women who engage in sexual intercourse at an early age and with multiple sex partners are at increased risk of developing dysplasia and cervical cancer. Carcinogens taken in with tobacco use are concentrated in the cervical mucous, predisposing users to development of cervical dysplasia and carcinoma. Although infection with syphilis necessitates screening for other sexually transmitted diseases and increases the likelihood that this patient may have an abnormal cytologic smear by virtue of increasing risk of having herpes simplex virus (HSV), it is not an independent risk factor for dysplasia.

**Characteristics of a screening test** • For a test to be useful in screening a large number of patients, it must have several characteristics. It should be relatively inexpensive, and available to a large number of patients and practitioners. It should be easy to perform and have good consistency among those interpreting results. It must have a high *sensitivity* (percentage of patients with disease having a positive result), so that few patients with the disease are missed (a low false negative rate). To compensate for this, there should be a follow-up test that is diagnostic and has high specificity. Screening tests themselves do not allow one to make a diagnosis because of the low specificity rate. The *disease* being tested should have a high prevalence in the population, and treatment of the disease early should decrease the incidence of more serious late sequelae. The Pap smear for cervical neoplasia satisfies these requirements. The diagnostic test for neoplasia is colposcopy with biopsy, and the serious late complication is cervical cancer.

**Pap smear frequency** • Pap smears should be performed on women annually after the age of 18 or when they become sexually active, whichever comes first. In the low-risk patient, this can be spaced out to every 1 to 3 years after three consecutive negative values have been obtained. High-risk patients that should always have annual screening include those with a history of a sexually transmitted disease, multiple sex partners, prior abnormal cytology, smokers, and patients with HIV.

**Cervical cancer screening** • The region of the cervix at greatest risk of undergoing neoplastic change is the transformation zone. These cells are initially columnar epithelium, but as the cervix evolutes, cells are exposed to bacteria, lower pH (about 4.5 to 5.0), and other harsh environmental factors of the vagina, and they undergo metaplasia to squamous epithelium.

Over 70 subtypes of HPV have been identified. A few of these are known to be associated with a higher risk of neoplastic change, including 16, 18, and 31. Other types are associated with development of genital warts. However, the presence of warts cannot provide reassurance that a high-risk type of HPV is not present, since any one patient may be infected with multiple subtypes simultaneously. At present, DNA typing of HPV is not part of screening for cervical cancer. Its role in managing high-risk patients is still being defined.

Cells can be obscured from adequate visualization by mucous and other debris. These samples are classified as "unsatisfactory" and should be repeated. This designation does not suggest atypical cells.

Annual Pap smear testing decreases a woman's risk of dying from cervical cancer from approximately 4 in 1000 to 5 in 10,000, a 90% reduction.

**Answers** • 1-C 2-B 3-E 4-E

## CASE PRESENTATION

A 50-year-old G3P3 presents with the complaint of increasing frequency of urination and episodes of "loss of urine." She often feels the sensation to void but when arriving to the restroom voids a minimal amount of urine. She does report nocturia, voiding four times each night. She has no significant past medical history and has been screened for diabetes mellitus, which was normal. She has had no surgeries. Her obstetrical history is significant for three spontaneous vaginal deliveries. A urinalysis is performed, which returns negative for blood, leukocytes, nitrites, protein, and glucose. Her pelvic exam reveals a normal vagina with no discharge; parous cervix without lesions; and uterus small, mobile, nontender, anteverted, with no adnexal masses. There is no evidence of a rectocele. A first-degree cystocele is noted.

1. The most likely diagnosis after taking the patient's history and physical is:
   A. Genuine stress incontinence
   B. Urge incontinence
   C. Overflow incontinence
   D. Chronic urinary tract infection
   E. None of the above
2. The etiology of this diagnosis is most likely:
   A. Resistant bacteria
   B. Detrusor muscle instability
   C. Anatomic change in urethrovesical angle
   D. Neurologic deficit
   E. None of the above
3. Which of the following tests would be most helpful in solidifying your diagnosis?
   A. Simple cystometrogram
   B. Repeat urine cultures every 6 weeks
   C. Q-tip test
   D. Cough stress test
   E. None of the above
4. Which of the following would be the treatment of choice?
   A. Nitrofurantoin
   B. Tolterodine
   C. Intermittent catheterization
   D. Bladder neck suspension
   E. None of the above
5. If the same patient presented to you with the complaint of increasing loss of urine with jogging or coughing, the etiology would be:
   A. Resistant bacteria
   B. Detrusor muscle instability
   C. Anatomic change in urethrovesical angle
   D. Neurologic deficit
   E. None of the above

## COMMENT

**Findings associated with urge incontinence** • Incontinence, or involuntary loss of urine, can be due to multiple etiologies. Genuine stress incontinence is characterized by involuntary loss of urine with increased intra-abdominal pressure such as coughing or sneezing. Overflow incontinence simply implies a hypotonic bladder, usually caused by a neurologic etiology. This may be due to chronic illness such as diabetes or from trauma resulting in lower motor neuron or spinal cord damage. This patient has textbook characteristics of urge incontinence. There is the increased sensation or "urge" to urinate, but little urine is expressed when trying to void. Also, due to the increased sensation to void, nocturia is a common complaint.

**Etiology of urge incontinence** • Urination is under voluntary control of the detrusor muscle of the bladder. Urge incontinence is caused by overactivity or "instability" of the detrusor muscle.

**Diagnostic tests** • A simple cystometrogram would be the most helpful test because it will identify detrusor instability. A simple cystometrogram can be performed in the office setting using a red rubber catheter with a 60-cc syringe attached. The catheter is placed in the urethra, and the bladder is filled with normal saline. During filling of the bladder, the patient is asked to cough. With irregular detrusor contractions the meniscus of the saline will move upward slightly after the cough. The Q-tip test is used to identify an anatomic change in the urethrovesical junction. A cotton-tip applicator is placed at the urethrovesical junction and the patient is asked to perform a Valsalva maneuver. The normal change in angle of the applicator is 30 degrees. A greater degree of angulation suggests an anatomic change in the urethra. The cough stress test also identifies genuine stress incontinence. The bladder is filled with normal saline and the patient is asked to cough. Involuntary spurts of urine suggest stress incontinence. A urine culture is performed during the incontinence workup, but repeated cultures are unnecessary.

**Treatment options** • Tolterodine would be the treatment of choice because this drug is an anticholinergic. Its mechanism of action is to inhibit the cholinergically innervated detrusor muscle. Nitrofurantoin is an antibiotic used for treatment of urinary tract infections. Intermittent catheterization is used for overflow incontinence to avoid overdistension. Bladder neck suspension by surgical intervention would be indicated for stress urinary incontinence.

**Genuine stress incontinence** • Involuntary loss of urine with cough or sneeze is characteristic of genuine stress urinary incontinence. Due to a change in the anatomic location of the urethra caused by pelvic relaxation, the intra-abdominal pressure from coughing exceeds the urethral pressure, thus leading to leakage of urine. This can be corrected by surgical correction of the urethrovesical junction. Examples of surgical procedures include retropubic urethropexy, needle suspension, and urethral sling.

**Answers** • 1-B 2-B 3-A 4-B 5-C

## CASE PRESENTATION

A 36-year old G1P1 presents to your office for her routine annual health maintenance exam. She has no complaints. She and her husband have been using condoms and she wishes to discuss other forms of contraception. Her past medical history is significant for tonsillectomy as a child. She has smoked one pack of cigarettes per day for 16 years. She has always had normal cervical cytology on Pap smear. She denies any history of sexually transmitted diseases. Her menstrual history is significant for bleeding every 28 days, 6 days in length. She denies dysmenorrhea. Her physical exam is without significant findings. Blood pressure is 120/78. Pelvic exam reveals normal external female genitalia; no vaginal discharge; cervix without lesions; uterus normal size, nontender, anteverted, mobile with no masses.

1. Which of the following forms of contraception is contraindicated for this patient?
   - A. IM medroxyprogesterone
   - B. Intrauterine device (IUD)
   - C. Diaphragm
   - D. Oral contraceptive pills
   - E. None of the above
2. Which of the following forms of contraception has the highest failure rate?
   - A. IM medroxyprogesterone
   - B. Intrauterine device
   - C. Diaphragm
   - D. Oral contraceptive pills
   - E. Each has an identical failure rate
3. Which of the following is an action of oral contraceptive pills causing contraception?
   - A. Alteration of cervical mucus
   - B. Inhibition of ovulation
   - C. Alteration of endometrium not conducive to implantation
   - D. All of the above
   - E. None of the above
4. Which of the following would deter you from recommending an IUD?
   - A. A patient with one mutually monogamous partner
   - B. A patient wishing to not have another child for more than 5 years
   - C. A patient with heavy menses
   - D. A patient with a recently treated episode of *Chlamydia* infection
   - E. All of the above
5. Which of the following would not be recommended for a patient with clinical depression?
   - A. IM medroxyprogesterone
   - B. Bilateral tubal ligation
   - C. Diaphragm placement
   - D. Condom use
   - E. None of the above

## COMMENT

**Smoking and oral contraceptives** • Because this patient is over 35 years of age and a smoker, oral contraceptives containing estrogen and progesterone are contraindicated. This contraindication is based on studies that have shown a dramatic increase in the incidence of cardiovascular events (myocardial infarction) in smokers over 35 years of age taking oral contraceptive pills. Due to the mortality associated with these events, other options should be used.

**Efficacy of contraception** • No method of birth control is 100% effective except for abstinence. All of the choices listed are adequate forms of birth control; however, due to patient compliance and imperfect use, failure rates exist. Failure rate indicates the chance of pregnancy within the first year of use. The failure rate of oral contraceptive pills with "perfect" use may be quoted as 0.1%. However, due to patients forgetting dosages, the "typical" failure rate is 3%. IM medroxyprogesterone (Depo-Provera) has a failure rate of 0.3%, while an IUD failure rate is quoted as approximately 1%. The diaphragm has the most varied results. With perfect use the failure rate resulting in pregnancy is approximately 6%, while the typical-use failure rate is 15% to 18%. This failure rate has been attributed to improper fitting, incorrect insertion, and lack of spermicide. The diaphragm should be inserted several hours prior to intercourse and should remain in place at least 6 hours after intercourse.

**Mechanism of action of oral contraceptives** • Oral contraceptives result in contraception by all the methods listed. Suppression of the luteinizing hormone surge inhibits ovulation. Thickening of the cervical mucus makes sperm penetration less likely. The level of estrogen and progesterone place the endometrium in a state in which implantation can not occur.

**Contraindications for IUD placement** • Intrauterine devices are now becoming a more common choice of contraception. Their popularity waned in the 1970s when the FDA, due to increased rates of pelvic infection, discontinued brands. There are two IUDs currently on the market: the Mirena, a 5-year levonorgestrel-containing IUD, and the ParaGuard T Copper, whose duration is 10 years. The IUD is a good choice for the mutually monogamous couple who are not planning to conceive for a long period of time. Heavy menses should not deter using an IUD because the progesterone-containing IUD may help alleviate this symptom. A patient with a known pelvic infection would not be a candidate for IUD placement due to possible ascension of bacteria leading to endometritis as well as salpingo-oophoritis. Infection and inflammation of pelvic organs may lead to scarring or adhesive disease, resulting in infertility and pelvic pain.

**Progestins and depression** • Patients with depression may be sensitive to large doses of progestins. A known side effect of progestins may be moodiness and depressed feelings. Of the choices listed, the IM medroxyprogesterone is the method containing the largest dose of progestin. Occasionally, a patient will also be sensitive to certain progestins in oral contraceptive pills. Before proceeding with a bilateral tubal ligation, a patient must understand that the procedure is a permanent sterilization. Studies have shown that a large percentage of patients who proceed with bilateral tubal ligation in their 20s have a high percentage of regret.

**Answers** • 1-D 2-C 3-D 4-D 5-A

## CASE PRESENTATION

A 30-year-old white G0P0 presents to your office complaining of diffuse cramping pain in her abdomen. The pain is worse with intercourse and occasionally with bowel movements. She denies nausea or vomiting. The pain is not associated with eating. She denies anorexia. Her last menstrual period was approximately 1 month prior to this visit, and she reports the pain was worse with menses. Her abdomen is soft, nontender, and nondistended with normoactive bowel sounds. Her pelvic exam reveals no vaginal discharge or cervical motion tenderness Her uterus is normal size, slightly fixed, retroverted, and diffusely tender. No adnexal masses are appreciated.

1. After taking the patient's history and physical, which would you order first?
   A. Pelvic ultrasound
   B. Urine βhCG
   C. Direct bilirubin
   D. KUB/abdominal series
   E. None of the above
2. Upon completion of the patient's history and physical, your preliminary diagnosis is which of the following?
   A. Appendicitis
   B. Acute cervicitis
   C. Small-bowel obstruction
   D. Endometriosis
   E. None of the above
3. Which of the following would be your first choice as a method of treatment?
   A. IM injection of ceftriaxone
   B. Laparotomy
   C. Oral contraceptive pills
   D. NPO with nasogastric tube placed
   E. None of the above
4. The patient has improvement in her pain with treatment. She wishes to discuss other possible outcomes or side effects of her diagnosis. Which of the following should be addressed?
   A. Possible decreased fertility
   B. Dyspareunia
   C. Possible change in bowel habits
   D. None of the above
   E. All of the above
5. The patient presents 12 months later with recurrence of pain and desires no medical management. Upon performing laparoscopy, what finding would you most likely encounter?
   A. Pus-filled fluid in cul-de-sac
   B. Torsion of ovary
   C. Gangrenous appendix
   D. Blue-brown "power burns" on ovaries
   E. All of the above

**Answers** • 1-B 2-D 3-C 4-E 5-D

## COMMENT

**Pelvic pain in a reproductive-aged woman** • No contraceptive history was taken in this sexually active patient. With abdominal pain and menses more than 1 month ago, urine βhCG would be most beneficial to aid in the diagnosis of a life-threatening problem such as an ectopic pregnancy. If the βhCG were positive, an ultrasound would be helpful in differentiating between an intrauterine pregnancy and an ectopic pregnancy. A direct bilirubin level is often elevated in a patient with cholelithiasis. Symptoms associated with cholelithiasis include right upper quadrant pain associated with eating. Abdominal exam will reveal a positive Murphy's sign: pain to palpation in right upper quadrant with inspiration. Radiological studies such as the KUB would be beneficial if small-bowel obstruction were suspected. Small-bowel obstruction often presents with nausea, vomiting, and abdominal distension. Bowel sounds may be absent or high pitched. Previous abdominal surgery is a significant risk factor for small-bowel obstruction.

**Signs and symptoms of endometriosis** • Reports of diffuse, severe pain coinciding with menses should immediately bring endometriosis to mind. Endometriosis often causes painful intercourse due to endometrial implants in the cul-de-sac and on the uterosacral ligaments and ovaries. Dyschezia (painful bowel movements) and dysuria may not be uncommon if there is bowel or bladder involvement. Appendicitis or small-bowel obstruction is not a likely choice, as the patient has a normal abdominal exam and no fever, nausea, vomiting, or anorexia. Cervicitis is unlikely with no complaint of vaginal discharge or cervical motion tenderness found on pelvic exam.

**Medical management** • Endometriosis is defined as endometrial stroma and glands found outside the uterus. The exact etiology is unknown. Theories of endometriosis origin include retrograde menstruation, hematogenous and lymphatic spread, and transformation of coelomic epithelium into endometrial type tissue. Treatment for endometriosis may be divided into medical and surgical treatments. Medical treatments focus on decreasing or ceasing menstruation. Oral contraceptive pills are considered the first line of therapy. Intramuscular medroxyprogesterone and gonadotropin-releasing hormone agonists also are used to induce a state of amenorrhea. Danazol is rarely used due to its androgenic, virilizing side effects. Danazol produces a low-estrogen, high-androgen environment that does not allow growth of endometriosis and also induces a state of amenorrhea.

**Side effects associated with endometriosis** • Patients with endometriosis may present with difficulty trying to conceive. The exact reason for infertility remains the subject of debate. Infertility may be due to endometriosis causing adhesions or anatomic distortion; however, infertility is also seen in patients with endometriosis with no evidence of adhesive disease. Endometriosis is not limited to gynecologic structures. Ureteral, bladder, and bowel/rectal involvement have been reported, with resulting pain on urination and defecation. Dyspareunia (pain with intercourse) may be caused by endometriosis implants on uterosacral ligaments, adhesions, and a severely retroverted uterus.

**Surgical management** • If medical therapy has failed, surgical management via laparoscopy is the next option. The pathognomonic characteristic seen upon visualizing the pelvis are endometrial implants most commonly found on the ovaries. Endometrial implants typically have a bluish-black appearance referred to as "powder burns." Other common areas of implants include the pouch of Douglas and uterosacral ligaments. Surgical management includes fulguration by cautery, laser, or resection of the endometriosis implants. More radical surgical management would include hysterectomy with bilateral salpingo-oophorectomy.

## CASE PRESENTATION

The pathology report of a 35-year-old smoker comes across your desk showing low-grade cervical intraepithelial neoplasia. She has never had an abnormal Pap smear. You check your last notes, and see that when you saw her, she was without complaints. She is monogamous with her husband but reports 15 lifetime partners. Her exam was normal; the cervix did not have any visible lesion, and was not friable.

1. Which of the following is an absolute indication for colposcopy?
   A. Atypical squamous cells of undetermined significance (ASCUS) in a patient with a history of normal Pap smears
   B. Unsatisfactory Pap smear
   C. Benign cervical changes on Pap smear
   D. High-grade squamous intraepithelial lesion (HGSIL) on Pap smear
   E. History of cervical cancer, treated with radical hysterectomy
2. Which of the following is not a part of a standard colposcopic examination?
   A. Speculum examination of the cervix under magnification
   B. Application of acetic acid to the cervix
   C. Biopsy of suspicious lesions
   D. Endocervical curettage
   E. Endometrial biopsy
3. Colposcopy shows a white lesion when exposed to acetic acid. Biopsy of the lesion returns cervical intraepithelial neoplasia type I (CIN I). Endocervical curettage is negative. The most appropriate management would be:
   A. Observation with repeat pap smear in 6 months
   B. Cryocautery
   C. Loop excision of the transformational zone (LETZ) (also known as loop electrocautery excision procedure, LEEP)
   D. Cold-knife conization (CKC)
   E. Hysterectomy
4. Which of the following would qualify colposcopy as "inadequate"?
   A. The entire transformational zone is seen.
   B. No lesion is seen, despite the abnormal Pap smear.
   C. The lesion is larger than 1 cm, but is seen completely.
   D. The lesion dives into the endocervical canal and is not seen in its entirety.
   E. The squamocolumnar junction is completely seen.
5. Which of the following is an indication for cervical conization by LETZ or CKC?
   A. CIN II lesion on the ectocervix
   B. Atypia within a sample from the endocervical curettage
   C. Pap smear showing CIN II but biopsy showing CIN I
   D. Recurrence of ectocervical disease after previous cryocautery

**Answers** • 1-D 2-E 3-B 4-D 5-B

## COMMENT

**Indications for colposcopy** • The predominant terminology for characterization of abnormal cytology is the Bethesda system. This system designates two categories: low-grade squamous intraepithelial lesions (LGSIL), which include cervical intraepithelial neoplasia I (CIN I); and high-grade squamous intraepithelial lesions (HGSIL), which include CIN II and III. Both LGSIL and HGSIL require examination with colposcopy and biopsies as indicated (though some argue that LGSIL can be observed). An ASCUS Pap result should be repeated in 4 to 6 months, and colposcopy performed only if the next result is abnormal (ASCUS or worse). Patients treated for cervical cancer can be followed with a Pap smear, and biopsies taken if lesions are seen or the Pap smear shows atypical cells. An "unsatisfactory" Pap smear should be repeated in 1 to 3 months.

**Procedure of colposcopy** • With colposcopy, the cervix (and vagina if necessary) is examined under high magnification with a powerful light source. The cervix is first prepared by soaking in acetic acid, which causes epithelial cells with a high nuclear to cytoplasmic ratio to appear white. Termed *acetowhite epithelium*, these are areas that should be targeted for biopsy. Usually an *endocervical curettage* (ECC) is performed with colposcopy to obtain a biopsy specimen from the endocervical canal, since this area cannot be visualized. An endometrial biopsy should be considered after an atypical glandular cell of undetermined significance (AGCUS) Pap, but is not a routine part of colposcopy.

**Treatment of visible CIN I** • Low-grade lesions on the ectocervix can be treated with cryocautery, with a 95% cure rate. Cryocautery involves freezing with liquid nitrogen passed through a metal tip that is applied to the cervix for 3 minutes, then off for 5 minutes, then on for another 3 minutes. Observation is the less preferable but reasonable option in a reliable patient who understands that progression is a possibility. In fact, about 65% of CIN I lesions will regress spontaneously, about 20% will not change, and about 15% will progress to more severe dysplasia.

Conization with LETZ or CKC is indicated if disease in the canal is suspected. A hysterectomy is usually only appropriate in women beyond their childbearing years with multiple episodes of neoplasia refractory to conservative treatment.

**Inadequate colposcopy** • For thorough colposcopic examination, four criteria must be met. The examiner must see (1) the entire lesion (if one is present), (2) the entire transformational zone, (3) the junction of the original squamous epithelium, and (4) the squamocolumnar junction. These qualifications satisfy the examiner that unseen disease in the endocervical canal does not exist. Absence of a lesion does not make colposcopy inadequate; the false positive rate of Pap smears is about 10% to 15%.

**Indications for conization** • The LETZ and CKC procedures are used to excise disease further in the endocervical canal. This is most commonly necessary when the endocervical curettage is positive. It is also indicated if the entire lesion cannot be seen, since cryotherapy would not be expected to reach the unseen part of the lesion. If the Pap smear indicates a higher grade of disease than is seen on biopsy by two levels (i.e., CIN III on Pap but CIN I on biopsy), the canal must be sampled to exclude the presence of unbiopsied CIN III in the endocervix. If an invasive neoplasm is suspected, a conization is needed to evaluate the depth of invasion, since depth of invasion dictates whether simple or radical hysterectomy is needed.

As long as recurrent low-grade disease is on the ectocervix, retreatment with cryocautery is appropriate.

## CASE PRESENTATION

An 18-year-old G1P0 with a 37 2/7 weeks' intrauterine pregnancy (IUP) presents to your office for a routine follow-up visit. Her only complaint is new onset indigestion. She denies vaginal bleeding, loss of fluid, or recent contractions. She reports good fetal movement. She denies headache or visual changes. Upon exam her fundal height is 30 cm. Lower extremity reflexes are 3+ bilaterally with 1+ pitting edema. Cervical exam is 1 centimeter dilated, 30% effaced and −2 station. Her blood pressure is 162/110. Urine dip reveals 3+ protein. A nonstress test (NST) is performed. The NST is reactive with fetal heart tones in the 130s. Tocometer reveals no uterine contractions.

1. Which of the following is the most likely diagnosis?
   A. Chronic hypertension
   B. Substance abuse
   C. Preeclampsia
   D. Molar pregnancy
   E. Gastroesophageal reflux disease
2. Which of the following tests would be *least* helpful in solidifying the final diagnosis?
   A. Aspartate aminotransferase (AST)
   B. Lactic dehydrogenase
   C. Platelet count
   D. Urine drug screen
   E. Uric acid
3. The laboratory tests return as follows: AST, 75 IU/L; creatinine, 0.9 mg/dL; platelets, 102; urine drug screen, negative; and uric acid, 6.2 mg/dL. What is the treatment of choice?
   A. Extended fetal monitoring on labor and delivery unit
   B. Induction of labor with Pitocin or prostaglandin
   C. Emergent cesarean section
   D. Follow-up in 1 week at physician's office
   E. All are acceptable treatment options
4. Which of the following clinical findings is the most worrisome regarding fetal well-being?
   A. Hyperreflexia
   B. Proteinuria
   C. Lagging fundal height
   D. Lower extremity pitting edema
   E. Facial and hand edema

## COMMENT

**Clinical findings associated with preeclampsia** • The most likely diagnosis of a primigravida with signs and symptoms of elevated blood pressure, proteinuria, edema, and hyperreflexia is preeclampsia. Preeclampsia is a hypertensive disease unique to pregnancy. It is typically noted in the third trimester and occurs more frequently in primigravidas. The etiology of preeclampsia is still not fully understood, although theories including vascular endothelial damage, abnormal placentation, and genetic predisposition have been proposed. Preeclampsia is divided into two categories, mild and severe. Mild preeclampsia is diagnosed by blood pressure greater than 140/90, 24-hour urine protein between 300 mg and 5 g, and edema. Criteria for severe preeclampsia include blood pressure greater than 160/110, 24-hour urine protein greater than 5 g, oliguria, CNS disturbances such as headache and scotomata, pulmonary edema, thrombocytopenia, and elevated liver function tests. Chronic hypertension is unlikely since this patient had no previous history of elevated blood pressures. Substance abuse, such as cocaine, may elevate blood pressure but would not produce proteinuria. Molar pregnancy is associated with elevated blood pressure and nausea but is diagnosed most often in the first trimester.

**Diagnostic tests** • With preeclampsia being the most obvious diagnosis, a urine drug test would not be helpful. HELLP syndrome (hemolysis, elevated liver enzymes, and low platelets) indicates the severe form of preeclampsia. Hemolysis is recognized by an abnormal peripheral blood smear and elevated lactic dehydrogenase. Liver enzymes, typically AST and alanine aminotransferase (ALT), are greater than 70 IU/L. Thrombocytopenia associated with HELLP syndrome is generally less than 100,000. A serum uric acid level less than 5 mg/dL is found in a normal pregnancy. Uric acid may be elevated in preeclampsia due to vasospasm and glomerular capillary endothelial swelling. Hemoglobin and hematocrit may be falsely elevated due to hemoconcentration encountered during preeclampsia.

**Treatment of preeclampsia** • The treatment for severe preeclampsia at any gestational age is delivery. Because the patient appears clinically stable, emergent cesarean is not indicated; induction with oxytocin or prostaglandins to obtain a vaginal delivery is reasonable. If the patient becomes unstable (i.e., inability to control blood pressures) or if the fetal status becomes nonreassuring, a cesarean section would be indicated. The management of mild preeclampsia at term is also delivery. Mild preeclampsia in the preterm patient may be managed with bed rest and close observation with fetal testing. If a patient is stable, she may be observed until term and then labor induced. If signs and symptoms of severe preeclampsia ensue during observation, then delivery is warranted. Because the greatest fear with preeclampsia is possible progression to eclampsia, seizure prophylaxis is administered during labor and 24 hours postpartum. The most common regimen is intravenous magnesium sulfate.

**Etiology of intrauterine growth restriction** • All of the findings listed may lead to the diagnosis of preeclampsia; however, lagging fundal height is the most worrisome finding listed. Lagging fundal height or size less than dates should make one suspicious of intrauterine growth restriction (IUGR). IUGR may be seen in patients with preeclampsia indicating poor placental perfusion. If this lagging fundal height is noted, ultrasound should be performed to estimate fetal weight. IUGR is defined as estimated fetal weight less than the tenth percentile for gestational age.

**Answers** • 1-C 2-D 3-B 4-C

## CASE PRESENTATION

A 55-year-old African American woman presents to your office for her annual health maintenance exam. She has been postmenopausal for approximately 6 years. She is not using hormone replacement therapy. She is currently taking prednisone 10 mg every day for rheumatoid arthritis. Her social history is significant for one pack of cigarettes per day for 30 years. She denies alcohol use. She does not have a daily exercise routine.

1. Which of the following is not a risk factor for osteoporosis when considering this patient?
   A. Thirty pack year smoker
   B. Daily corticosteroid use
   C. African American ethnicity
   D. Postmenopausal with no hormone replacement use
   E. All of the above are known risk factors
2. Which study is currently considered the gold standard to screen this patient for osteoporosis?
   A. Magnetic resonance imaging (MRI)
   B. X-ray of hip and spine
   C. Quantitative computed tomography (CT)
   D. Dual energy x-ray absorptiometry
   E. None of the above
3. The osteoporotic fracture attributing to the greatest mortality, cost, and loss of ability to perform activities of daily living is:
   A. Colles
   B. Hip
   C. Ankle
   D. Vertebral
   E. Humerus
4. This patient's screening test returns with evidence of osteoporosis. Which drug would be used as first-line therapy?
   A. Hormone replacement (estrogen and progesterone)
   B. Calcitonin
   C. Bisphosphonates
   D. Fluoride
   E. None of the above
5. Which of the following treatments for osteoporosis is the only drug that stimulates osteoblast activity?
   A. Hormone replacement therapy
   B. Calcitonin
   C. Parathyroid hormone
   D. Bisphosphonates
   E. All of the above

## COMMENT

**Risk factors associated with osteoporosis** • Menopause is a state of estrogen deficiency. This patient is taking no form of hormone replacement therapy, which places her at risk for osteoporosis. Smoking is a well-known risk factor because this habit may induce menopause at an earlier age. Chronic steroid use for rheumatoid arthritis, asthma, or other medical conditions should immediately raise suspicion for osteoporosis. Corticosteroids have a direct effect on bone, causing inhibition of bone formation by enhancing bone resorption. Women at highest risk for osteoporosis have been noted to be of Caucasian and Asian descent. Recent investigation has also shown Hispanic descent to be at risk. African Americans appear to have the lowest rate of osteoporosis. Other known risk factors include family history of osteoporosis and history of prior unexplained fracture.

**Diagnostic tests** • Dual energy x-ray absorptiometry, known as the DEXA scan, is now considered the gold standard for screening. MRI and quantitative CT have been shown to detect osteoporosis but are more costly. Plain films of spine and hip have not been proven to help predict or diagnose osteoporosis.

**Osteoporotic fractures** • Although vertebral fractures are the most common, hip fractures are generally the most debilitating, with a 24% mortality rate within the first year of occurrence. Also, these patients incur a large financial burden due to long-term nursing and medical care as well as family care and lost wages. Hip fracture patients also tend to have a great deal of pain and often suffer from depression due to inability to perform activities of daily living.

**Treatment options** • Even though new medications are available or currently evolving for the treatment of osteoporosis, first-line therapy continues to be hormone replacement therapy. Contraindications for estrogen use that should be considered include history of thrombosis such as deep venous thrombosis or cerebral vascular accident, liver disease, and unexplained vaginal bleeding. Calcitonin and bisphosphonates are also used in the treatment of osteoporosis by inhibiting osteoclast activity. Fluoride has been shown to stimulate osteoblasts, but the bone that is formed is structurally weak and may fracture.

**Mechanism of action** • Of the choices listed, parathyroid hormone is the only drug whose mechanism of action is to stimulate osteoblast function to create bone. Calcitonin, hormone replacement therapy, bisphosphonates, and raloxifene all work by inhibiting osteoclast activity, decreasing the resorption of bone.

**Answers** • 1-C 2-D 3-B 4-A 5-C

## CASE PRESENTATION

During her annual exam, a 16-year-old high school student reports that for the last 2 years her menses have become painful. The pain is described as cramping just over the symphysis pubis. This is associated with pressure, nausea, and diarrhea. Acetaminophen has given minimal improvement. She has noticed that her menses are more regular, whereas 2 years ago they were unpredictable in timing and duration. She denies vaginal discharge, fever, or pain between periods. She is not sexually active. A pelvic exam is completely normal. The pregnancy test and urinalysis are negative.

1. The working diagnosis should be:
   - A. Primary dysmenorrhea
   - B. Secondary dysmenorrhea
   - C. Endometriosis
   - D. Pelvic inflammatory disease
   - E. Ectopic pregnancy
2. The primary mechanism of primary dysmenorrhea is:
   - A. Release of an ovum from the ovary
   - B. Accumulation of fluid in the peritoneal cavity
   - C. Inflammatory reaction to blood in the uterine cavity
   - D. Non-neoplastic invasion of endometrial tissue into the myometrium
   - E. Prostaglandin production
3. The initial treatment should be:
   - A. Oral contraceptives
   - B. Gonadotropin-releasing hormone (GnRH) agonists
   - C. Nonsteroidal anti-inflammatory drugs (NSAIDs)
   - D. Mild narcotics
   - E. Cyclooxygenase-2 selective inhibitors

## COMMENT

**Definition of primary dysmenorrhea** • Primary dysmenorrhea is defined as painful menses without an underlying pathology. Secondary dysmenorrhea, on the other hand, has an underlying cause, such as endometriosis, obstruction, or infection. In this patient, there is no evidence on history or physical of an alternate etiology, and the history is consistent with primary dysmenorrhea.

Endometriosis is the most common cause of secondary dysmenorrhea. The classic triad is dysmenorrhea, dyspareunia, and infertility. The diagnosis of endometriosis can be suspected on history and physical examination, but can only be made by visual confirmation at the time of surgery, or pathologic diagnosis on a surgical specimen. Pelvic inflammatory disease should be accompanied by leukorrhea at the cervical os and cervical motion tenderness in a sexually active female. An ectopic pregnancy may cause pain, but not for 2 years, and is ruled out with a negative pregnancy test.

**Mechanism of primary dysmenorrhea** • The distinction that primary dysmenorrhea does not have an underlying etiology is something of a misnomer, because it is known to result from the effects of prostaglandins, primarily $PGF_{2\alpha}$. Prostaglandins are produced by *secretory* endometrium, and therefore only accompany ovulation. This explains the observation that dysmenorrhea is often minimal in the first few years of menstruation, when menses are usually anovulatory. The distinction of primary versus secondary dysmenorrhea can be suspected on history and physical, but it is technically a retrospective diagnosis because an underlying cause cannot be definitively excluded without an exhaustive workup.

Pain due to release of an ovum can be appreciated by some women. It is termed *mittelschmerz* and occurs at midcycle. Treatment is ovulation suppression. The presence of a significant amount of fluid in the abdominal cavity is abnormal and should prompt a search for a cause, such as bleeding from a ruptured cyst or pelvic inflammatory disease. Adenomyosis is a cause of secondary dysmenorrhea, usually in older women, and results from the invasion of non-neoplastic endometrium into the underlying myometrium, causing chronic pelvic pain and dysmenorrhea.

**Treatment of primary dysmenorrhea** • NSAIDs are the therapy of choice for primary dysmenorrhea. As prostaglandin inhibitors, they combat the pathophysiologic mechanism and are effective in 70% of cases. They may be initiated 1 to 2 days before anticipated menses for maximal effectiveness. Oral contraceptives are also a good choice, especially in women who need contraception or when NSAIDs only give partial relief. The combination of NSAIDs and oral contraceptives is effective in 90% of cases. If together they are inadequate, the diagnosis should be questioned and causes of secondary dysmenorrhea should be explored.

Cyclooxygenase-2 selective inhibitors have been approved for treatment of primary and secondary dysmenorrhea. However, given the added expense, they are best used in patients at risk for peptic ulcer disease. Narcotics are only appropriate for short courses in cases of severe dysmenorrhea until alternate therapies such as surgery are explored. GnRH agonists would relieve these symptoms by making the patient anovulatory, but their expense (on the order of $500 per month) and need for only short-term use (less than 1 year) make them inappropriate for treatment of primary dysmenorrhea.

**Answers** • 1-A 2-E 3-C

## CASE PRESENTATION

A 58-year-old woman presents complaining of vulvar itching for 1 month. She has been postmenopausal for 10 years and takes conjugated estrogen 0.625 mg and medroxyprogesterone acetate 5 mg daily. She has tried petroleum jelly and hydrocortisone cream 1% without relief. On exam, you notice a 1 cm by 1 cm lesion where the skin is broken, slightly erythematous, and friable on the inferior aspect of the right labia majora. The majority of the vulva has a thin, whitish appearance.

1. The next appropriate step should be:
   A. Reassurance and observation, with reexamination in 1 month
   B. Treatment with conjugated estrogen cream
   C. Punch biopsy of the lesion
   D. Simple excision of the lesion
   E. Wide excision with inguinal node dissection
2. If the lesion were biopsied and pathology results showed hyperkeratosis, a collagenous-like material beneath the epithelium, and chronic inflammation, consistent with lichen sclerosis, which of the following would be the most appropriate treatment?
   A. 2% testosterone cream twice daily
   B. 1% hydrocortisone daily
   C. 0.05% clobetasol twice daily
   D. 2% progesterone cream
   E. Simple excision
3. If the biopsy results showed vulvar intraepithelial neoplasia with severe dysplasia, the treatment of choice would be:
   A. Observation with repeat biopsy if the lesion does not resolve spontaneously
   B. Laser ablation of the lesion
   C. Simple excision
   D. Wide local excision
   E. Radical local excision with ipsilateral inguinal node dissection

## COMMENT

**Biopsy of vulvar lesion** • Any new vulvar lesion in a postmenopausal woman should be biopsied to exclude malignancy. This also applies to younger women in whom the diagnosis is not certain or whose lesion does not respond to appropriate treatment. Vulvar itching is the most common symptom of both vulvar intraepithelial neoplasia and vulvar cancer.

The epithelium of the vagina may become thin and pruritic in the postmenopausal patient. Although oral estrogens are effective in some cases, the addition of conjugated estrogen cream is sometimes necessary. The vulva, however, does not respond to such treatment. A biopsy should be obtained before simple excision is performed, since more extensive excision is necessary if the lesion is malignant. Wide excision with inguinal node dissection is needed for vulvar cancer, but this is inappropriate without a certain diagnosis.

**Management of lichen sclerosis** • Lichen sclerosis is the most common white lesion of the vulva. Its diagnosis is suggested by a vulvar appearance of thin, white epithelium, often compared to cigarette paper. Biopsy confirms the diagnosis, and is usually indicated at initial presentation to exclude vulvar intraepithelial neoplasia (VIN) and vulvar cancer. The treatment of choice used to be testosterone cream, but recent studies have shown clobetasol, a high-dose steroid, to be more effective, with an 80% resolution rate (compared to 50% for testosterone cream). The suggested regimen is application twice daily for 1 month, daily for 2 months, then taper to an intermediate steroid cream. Recurrence is common, requiring chronic treatment in most patients.

**Management of vulvar intraepithelial neoplasia and vulvar cancer** • Surgical excision is the preferred treatment of vulvar neoplasia. This allows pathologic examination to exclude a focus of malignancy in the lesion. A disease-free border of at least 5 mm constitutes a wide excision, and is preferred. A simple excision (removal of just the lesion) increases the risk of positive margins and recurrence.

Observation is inappropriate in this neoplastic process because spontaneous resolution is uncommon and a malignancy cannot be excluded. After an initial excision, observation can be considered with low-grade lesions in patients who can be closely followed. Laser ablation is sometimes employed in multifocal lesions in which surgical excision would have to be extensive. This is preferably employed in mildly dysplastic lesions that have recurred, in which malignancy has been excluded with an initial surgical excision. Sometimes the two modalities can be used in combination, with excision of the portion most suspicious for possible malignancy, and laser ablation of the remaining tissue. An inguinal lymph node dissection is indicated for vulvar cancer.

**Answers** • 1-C 2-C 3-D

## CASE PRESENTATION

A 25-year-old G2P1 with a 35 2/7 weeks' intrauterine pregnancy presents to the emergency room by ambulance after a motor vehicle accident. The patient was an unrestrained driver. A vehicle traveling approximately 55 miles per hour hit her car in the driver's door. The patient reports hitting the steering wheel with her head but did not lose consciousness. She has no known medical history. Her obstetrical history is significant for one term spontaneous vaginal delivery 3 years ago. She has received prenatal care throughout this pregnancy and thus far has been uneventful. She does report abdominal cramping that is increasing in severity and thinks the fetus has not moved. She denies loss of amniotic fluid. Upon exam her vitals are blood pressure 90/60, pulse 114, respirations 22. Fundal height is 35 cm, abdomen is tense and distended. Cervix on examination is closed, 2 cm long, high. There is a significant amount of bright red blood in the vagina. Her left femur and ankle appear fractured, but the patient continues to have good pulses and sensation.

1. After performing the patient's history and physical, you are most concerned about:
   A. Preterm labor
   B. Placenta previa
   C. Preeclampsia
   D. Abruptio placenta
   E. All of the above
2. Which of the following would be the last action you would perform regarding her workup?
   A. Type and cross pack red blood cells
   B. Large-bore IV placement
   C. CT of abdomen and pelvis
   D. Doppler of fetal heart tones
   E. All of these could be performed simultaneously
3. Which of the following would be the best next step?
   A. Orthopedic surgery of ankle and femur
   B. IV magnesium tocolysis
   C. Induction of labor with IV oxytocin
   D. Cesarean section
   E. None of the above
4. Which of the following is the mechanism of action for this patient's diagnosis?
   A. Sheering of the placenta from the uterine wall
   B. Implantation of the placenta through the myometrium
   C. Infectious
   D. Idiopathic
   E. None of the above
5. Upon discharge from the hospital, which lab test must be reviewed?
   A. Rh status
   B. Rubella
   C. Rapid plasma reagent (RPR)
   D. Hepatitis B surface antigen
   E. None of the above

## COMMENT

**Trauma in the pregnant patient** • A pregnant patient involved in a motor vehicle accident presenting with abdominal pain, vaginal bleeding, and deteriorating vitals signs must have the presumed diagnosis of abruptio placenta. With the possibility of rapid blood loss and resulting coagulopathy, maternal and fetal mortality is high without rapid intervention. Placental abruption can range from slight vaginal bleeding with normal maternal and fetal status to severe bleeding, uterine tetany, and maternal and fetal distress. Placenta previa often causes vaginal bleeding, but is described as painless bleeding. Severe preeclampsia may cause bleeding due to low platelets and coagulopathy but there is no evidence of other associated symptoms such as elevated blood pressures, CNS symptoms, or edema. Preterm labor is unlikely because the patient does not describe regular uterine contractions and the cervix has no evidence of dilatation.

**Making the diagnosis quickly** • Because abruptio placenta is the presumed diagnosis, time is of essence. Due to the amount of blood loss that may occur, placing an intravenous line for fluid resuscitation and ensuring availability of blood products are imperative. Fetal Doppler or ultrasound is imperative to assess heart tone and fetal viability. Because abruptio placenta is the most life-threatening diagnosis, proceeding with CT of the abdomen for other etiology of bleeding and abdominal pain would be incorrect. Her orthopedic injury should be evaluated after she is stabilized.

**Treatment of placental abruption** • Due to the urgent nature of this case the only feasible answer is to proceed with an emergency cesarean section. Tocolysis for preterm labor is not indicated, and vaginal induction would entail too much time before delivery of the fetus.

**Etiology of abruption** • Abruptio placenta is the premature separation or sheering of the placenta away from its vascular supply of the placental wall. In this patient the etiology is due to blunt trauma. The patient was an unrestrained driver encountering a large impact at a high rate of speed. A lap and shoulder belt are advocated for pregnant drivers. Other etiologies associated with abruptio placenta include chronic hypertension, cocaine abuse, and rapid decompression of an overdistended uterus seen with polyhydramnios. Placenta previa is due to implantation of the placenta into the myometrium of the uterus. Preterm labor is often due to infectious or idiopathic reasons.

**Preventing isoimmunization** • After any case where maternal-fetal blood exchange may have occurred, the Rh status must be checked. If Rh is found to be negative Rh immune globulin should be administered to prevent isoimmunization in future pregnancies. Other indications include amniocentesis, vaginal delivery, cesarean section, spontaneous and elective abortions, external cephalic version, and ectopic pregnancies. Although the other prenatal lab tests are important, it would not be imperative to check these before discharge.

**Answers** • 1-D 2-C 3-D 4-A 5-A

## CASE PRESENTATION

You are called to see a 30-year-old G3P0A2 woman who delivered a 39 6/7 weeks' infant by cesarean section approximately 28 hours ago. Her obstetrical history is significant for two first trimester spontaneous abortions. She presented to labor and delivery with regular uterine contractions and stated that her "water broke" sometime yesterday. She now has a temperature of 101.5° Fahrenheit. She did not have a fever during labor. Her labor was approximately 20 hours in duration. She progressed to 7 cm without difficulty. After numerous cervical checks, she had not changed in 4 hours. Cesarean section was performed for arrest of dilatation. She currently has no complaints. She has been ambulating, eating, and voiding without difficulty. She is breast-feeding. Her exam reveals regular heart rate and rhythm, chest clear to auscultation, with breasts nonengorged. Abdomen and fundus are tender to palpation with no rebound or guarding. A white count is ordered and returns as 18,000. Urinalysis is negative.

1. Which of the following should also be inspected carefully in this patient with postpartum fever?
   A. Tympanic membranes
   B. Oropharynx
   C. Costovertebral angles
   D. Bilateral extremities
   E. None of the above
2. What is your current working diagnosis for this patient?
   A. Appendicitis
   B. Nephrolithiasis
   C. Septic pelvic thrombosis
   D. Endometritis
   E. None of the above
3. Which of the following may be attributed to this patient's diagnosis?
   A. Prolonged rupture of membranes
   B. Numerous cervical exams
   C. Cesarean section
   D. All of the above
   E. None of the above
4. Which of the following would be the best treatment option?
   A. IV heparin challenge
   B. Dilatation and curettage
   C. Laparotomy
   D. Broad-spectrum antibiotics
   E. None of the above

## COMMENT

**Differential diagnoses** • Because pregnancy is a hypercoagulable state and because this patient is postoperative from a surgery, a deep vein thrombosis should be in the differential diagnosis of postpartum fever. The classic appearance of a deep vein thrombosis is fever with an erythematous, edematous calf or thigh. Palpation may reveal a cord-like texture. Pain with flexion of the foot may accompany a deep vein thrombosis. This is known as Homans' sign. Deep vein thrombosis may be evaluated with ultrasound Dopplers of the veins. Although pharyngitis and otitis may cause fever, they would not be as highly suspected in the puerperium. Pregnant women do present with pyelonephritis as a source of fever, but the urinalysis for this patient was negative.

**Fundal tenderness** • A postpartum patient with fever greater than 100.4° Fahrenheit on two separate occasions within 24 hours or one temperature greater than 101.0° Fahrenheit should be examined. Common causes of postpartum fever that should be considered include pneumonia, wound infection, endomyometritis, deep vein thrombosis, breast engorgement or mastitis, medications, and pyelonephritis. With fever and fundal tenderness, the most obvious diagnosis is endomyometritis—infection of endometrium and myometrium. This patient has no symptoms of either nephrolithiasis or appendicitis. Septic pelvic thrombosis is often a diagnosis of exclusion in a postpartum patient when no other source is obvious.

**Risks factors associated with endometritis** • This patient presents with numerous reasons for postpartum endometritis. Prolonged rupture of membranes may allow the ascension of multiple vaginal flora organisms to the upper genital tract and peritoneal cavity. Because this patient was in labor for an extended period of time, multiple cervical exams were performed, which also increases access of vaginal flora. Finally, cesarean section places the patient at highest risk for infection. When cesarean section is performed after a prolonged labor with ruptured membranes, the incidence of endometritis is approximately 20%.

**Microbiology of endometritis** • The etiology of endomyometritis is a polymicrobial infection. Common offending organisms include *Escherichia coli*, *Klebsiella pneumoniae*, *Proteus* species, and *Prevotella* species. Antibiotics used should cover Gram-positive and Gram-negative organisms and anaerobes. Dilatation and curettage would be indicated if there was evidence of retained placenta, but retained placenta is usually accompanied with continued vaginal bleeding. Laparotomy is not indicated for a first-line treatment of endometritis. Intravenous heparin therapy is used in the diagnosis and treatment of septic pelvic thrombosis. In a patient with no other source of postpartum fever, a heparin challenge may be administered. If the patient defervesces, the diagnosis of septic pelvic thrombosis is made and heparin is continued for treatment of the thrombosis.

**Answers** • 1-D 2-D 3-B 4-D

## CASE PRESENTATION

A 34-year-old G3P2 with 37 4/7 weeks' intrauterine pregnancy presents to your office complaining of painful regular uterine contractions. She denies leakage of fluid or vaginal bleeding. She reports good fetal movement. She has had no problems throughout her pregnancy. Her obstetrical history is significant for two term spontaneous vaginal deliveries. She has an occasional asthma attack, which is relieved with an Albuterol inhaler. She also complains of "bumps" on her vulva that suddenly appeared. She has never noticed these before and complains that they are extremely painful. Exam reveals temperature of 98.4, blood pressure 118/78, pulse 76. Abdomen is nontender, gravid, with fundal height 38 cm. External genitalia exam reveals six to seven small, raised, erythematous vesicular lesions on bilateral labia majora. There is no vaginal discharge and cervix is 4/75%/−1. Fetal heart tones are in the 140s and reactive. Tocometer reveals contractions every 6 minutes.

1. After performing this patient's exam, what is the most likely diagnosis?
   A. Syphilis
   B. Herpes simplex virus
   C. Folliculitis
   D. Chancroid
   E. None of the above
2. Which test would most likely help solidify your diagnosis?
   A. Culture of the lesion
   B. Wet prep
   C. Punch biopsy
   D. Dark-field examination
   E. None of the above
3. Regarding the patient's pregnancy, which of the following would be your next step?
   A. Admit patient to labor and delivery and await spontaneous vaginal delivery
   B. Begin IV oxytocin for augmentation
   C. Send patient walking and repeat cervical check in 2 hours
   D. Proceed with cesarean section
   E. None of the above
4. If this patient had not shown evidence of labor, what would be the appropriate treatment?
   A. Cephalexin 500 mg orally four times a day for 7 days
   B. Benzathine penicillin G 2.4 million units IM
   C. Azithromycin 1000 mg orally and ceftriaxone 250 mg IM
   D. Valacyclovir 500 mg orally twice a day for 7 days
   E. None of the above
5. Which of the following is a condition in which this patient's diagnosis may be more prevalent?
   A. Renal transplant
   B. Pregnancy
   C. HIV infection
   D. All of the above
   E. None of the above

## COMMENT

**Physical findings associated with herpes** • The most common diagnosis in the United States of multiple, painful, raised vesicular vulvar lesions in a sexually active patient is herpes simplex virus (HSV). Two types of herpes simplex virus exist. These are referred to as type 1 and type 2. Type 1 is typically found in the oral region, while type 2 is found in the genital region. Chancroid is also painful, but is not common in the United States and often presents as a single, painful lesion. Folliculitis is infection and inflammation of hair follicles. Folliculitis may be moderately tender but is confined to areas of hair growth. Primary syphilis presents with nontender, painless lesions.

**Diagnostic tests** • The most helpful test would be culture of the lesion for the herpes virus. Chancroid's offending agent, *Haemophilus ducreyi,* may be cultured but requires a special media, which is not readily available in most laboratories. Dark-field examination is used to visualize *Treponema pallidum,* the spirochete responsible for syphilis. A punch biopsy would be extremely uncomfortable for this patient. Punch biopsies are performed when pathology is desired for questionable vulvar lesions.

**Management of labor with active herpes infection** • This patient is obviously in active labor with regular uterine contractions and cervical dilatation. Because this is the first painful outbreak this patient has reported, it should be considered as primary herpes. This is a worrisome condition because the rate of transmission of the herpes virus to the fetus with vaginal delivery is approximately 50%. With recurrent herpes the transmission is less than 5%. Passage of the herpes virus to the fetus with vaginal delivery may result in conditions such as meningitis and encephalitis. The mortality of infected neonates may reach 50% to 60%. With either a primary or recurrent HSV outbreak, the correct management is to proceed with cesarean section.

**Treatment options** • The treatment for an HSV outbreak is an antiviral. Of the options listed, valacyclovir 500 mg orally twice a day for 7 to 10 days is the treatment of choice. Other antivirals that may be used include acyclovir and famciclovir. Folliculitis is treated with warm sitz baths and an antibiotic that covers *Staphylococcus* and *Streptococcus* species, such as a cephalosporin. Chancroid requires IM ceftriaxone and oral azithromycin. Primary, secondary, or early latent syphilis is treated with IM penicillin G.

**Outbreaks in the immunosuppressed patient** • The herpes virus lies dormant in dorsal root ganglia. Increased emergence occurs in patients with conditions placing them in a state of immunosuppression. All of the conditions listed are considered states of immunosuppression and can be associated with increased HSV outbreaks.

**Answers** • 1-B 2-A 3-D 4-D 5-D

## CASE PRESENTATION

A 24-year-old woman now 2 weeks postpartum presents to your office with the complaint of subjective fever and chills for the past 2 days. She has been breast-feeding since delivery and is not supplementing with bottled formula. She states that her left breast is tender and firm. She denies nausea, vomiting, cough, or dysuria. Her temperature is 101.8, and upon inspection of the breast, the left breast is tender to touch with erythematous streaks. No obvious mass is palpated. There is no lymphadenopathy. The right breast is without significant findings.

1. The most likely diagnosis of this patient is:
   A. Mastitis
   B. Breast abscess
   C. Breast engorgement
   D. Normal findings of breast-feeding mother
   E. Intraductal papilloma
2. The most common pathogen responsible for this condition is:
   A. *Salmonella typhi*
   B. *Staphylococcus aureus*
   C. *Staphylococcus epidermidis*
   D. *Streptococcus pneumoniae*
   E. *Streptococcus viridans*
3. The patient has no known drug allergies. The treatment of choice is:
   A. Inpatient intravenous ampicillin
   B. Drainage of breast abscess
   C. Outpatient oral dicloxacillin
   D. Outpatient oral ofloxacin
   E. None of the above
4. Regarding breast-feeding, the patient should:
   A. Discontinue breast-feeding until infection has resolved
   B. Continue breast-feeding
   C. Begin bottle formula feedings
   D. Begin cup feeding
   E. None of the above

## COMMENT

**Diagnosis of mastitis** • A patient who complains of breast tenderness and fever when breast-feeding should be examined. Breast engorgement may cause discomfort and enlargement of the breasts but is usually accompanied by a low-grade fever (100.4° to 100.9°). Treatment may consist of ice packs and analgesics such as acetaminophen. A patient with an erythematous, tender breast, malaise, and fever of more than 101.0° should make one suspicious of mastitis. Mastitis is defined as inflammation of the lactiferous glands and ducts. A discrete mass palpated in an erythematous breast-feeding patient is most likely an abscess. Abscesses generally do not respond to antibiotic therapy and need drainage. Intraductal papilloma is a benign breast condition usually accompanied by spontaneous serosanguineous nipple discharge. No fever or erythema is noted. Treatment for these benign tumors is excision of the involved duct and surrounding tissue.

**Etiology of mastitis** • *Staphylococcus aureus* is responsible for approximately 40% of all cases of mastitis. Others include group A and B streptococci, *Haemophilus influenzae, Escherichia coli, Enterococcus faecalis, Enterobacter cloacae, Serratia marcescens,* and *Klebsiella pneumoniae.*

**Treatment of mastitis** • The treatment of choice for mastitis in a patient with no known drug allergies is oral dicloxacillin. Erythromycin or cephalosporin is the treatment of choice in penicillin-allergic patients. Hospitalization is usually unnecessary for the treatment of mastitis unless a patient is not responding to oral antibiotics or if there is suspicion of an abscess. Other palliative measures include acetaminophen, hydration, and ice packs to the breast.

**Breast-feeding with a known infection** • The patient should continue to breast-feed, because emptying the clogged and infected milk duct is needed. Suckling from an infected breast does not appear to cause adverse effects in the infant. Bottled formula feeding or cup feeding should not be instituted.

**Answers** • 1-A 2-B 3-C 4-B

## CASE PRESENTATION

A 32-year-old woman presents complaining of left pelvic discomfort since missing her menses 1 week ago. The pain is described as intermittently crampy with a dull ache the majority of the time. On exam she has a normal-sized uterus with fullness in the left adnexa, spanning approximately 5 cm, which is very mildly tender. The right adnexa is normal.

1. The most appropriate next step is:
   A. Pelvic ultrasound
   B. Pregnancy test
   C. Diagnostic laparoscopy
   D. Reexamine in 1 week
   E. Reexamine in 1 month
2. With a negative pregnancy test and a pelvic ultrasound showing a 4 cm by 5 cm simple cyst in the left adnexa, which of the following is true?
   A. She should be reexamined in 6 months.
   B. She should be reexamined after her next menses.
   C. The underlying pathology is ectopic implantation of endometrial tissue.
   D. The mass is probably a benign neoplasm.
   E. Surgical excision is indicated.
3. The most common ovarian neoplasm in all women is:
   A. Functional cyst
   B. Serous cystadenocarcinoma
   C. Serous cystadenoma
   D. Benign cystic teratoma
   E. Krukenberg tumor
4. In a 32-year-old patient with an 8-cm solid and cystic adnexal mass, ascites, and a right-sided pleural effusion, which of the following is true?
   A. If the cancer antigen 125 (CA125) level is 50 (normal, $<30$), the risk of ovarian cancer is about 90%.
   B. Surgical excision is not indicated.
   C. If pathology indicates a benign neoplasm, it is most likely a stromal cell neoplasm.
   D. The mass is probably functional, producing sex steroids.
   E. Ascites results from metastasis to the liver.

## COMMENT

**Ectopic pregnancy triad** • The most important pathology to exclude first is an ectopic pregnancy, suggested by the triad of amenorrhea, pelvic pain, and an adnexal mass. Ectopic pregnancies cause the deaths of approximately 30 to 40 women each year. Of these, an estimated 70% have seen a physician since complaints began.

**Management of a simple cyst** • A unilocular cyst in a reproductive-aged woman is most likely a functional cyst. There are two types: follicular and corpus luteal. Follicular cysts result from anovulation and continued growth of the follicle due to persistent secretion of estrogen by granulosa cells. Corpus luteal cysts normally occur after each ovulation, and may persist and enlarge. Functional cysts are not considered neoplasms. Because both of these cysts can be associated with missed menses, ectopic pregnancy is usually in the differential diagnosis. It may be impossible to determine which type the cyst is, but this does not matter because both types behave the same. Both types will resolve spontaneously, with the next menstrual cycle. Six months is too long a time to delay making a more specific diagnosis.

Although a benign neoplasm may have this appearance on ultrasound, 75% of palpable masses in *all* reproductive-aged women are functional cysts. Because most cystic masses will spontaneously resolve, surgical excision is only indicated if it does not spontaneously resolve, or becomes symptomatic (torsion, rupture, etc.). If a mass of 5 cm or greater persists, excision should be strongly considered to rule out a neoplasm and avoid morbidity from torsion. Endometriosis can be associated with an endometrioma (the so-called chocolate cyst), but these are filled with thick fluid, giving them a characteristic complex appearance on ultrasound.

**Most common ovarian neoplasms** • The benign cystic teratoma, also called a mature teratoma or dermoid, is the most common ovarian neoplasm in women. Although the functional cyst is the most common adnexal mass in women, it is not neoplastic in pathology. The serous cystadenocarcinoma is the most common *malignant* ovarian neoplasm in women. Its benign counterpart, the serous cystadenoma, is the most common *epithelial* ovarian tumor (of the three subtypes—epithelial, stromal, or germ cell—epithelial are the most common). Krukenberg ovarian tumors (malignant tumors metastatic to the ovary) represent 5% to 10% of all ovarian malignancies.

**Meigs' syndrome** • In a patient with a pelvic mass and ascites, excision is indicated to exclude a malignancy. Although an elevated CA125 level would make a malignancy more likely, a normal level is not helpful, since not all ovarian malignancies produce CA125. In fact, of all early (stage I) cancers, 50% have a normal CA125. In ovarian neoplasms, ascites results from two processes, often in combination: increased production of serosal fluid by the neoplasm, which increases with surface area; and obstruction of peritoneal fluid reuptake by lymphatic tissue due to metastatic nodal disease. The ovarian fibroma is a benign stromal ovarian neoplasm that represents only 10% of all neoplasms. In this scenario, however, it would be the most likely lesion if it were benign, because of its solid components, age of the patient, and associated findings. The triad of benign ovarian fibroma, ascites, and hydrothorax is known as Meigs' syndrome. The fibroma is the only one of the stromal neoplasms that is not functional. Granulosa theca cell tumors primarily produce estrogenic steroids. Sertoli-Leydig cell tumors primarily produce androgenic steroids, often leading to masculinization.

**Answers** • 1-B 2-B 3-D 4-C

## CASE PRESENTATION

A 28-year-old G3P2 at 38 5/7 weeks' gestation presents with regular uterine contractions and cervical change to 5 centimeters. Her antepartum course has been complicated by poorly controlled gestational diabetes, with a recent ultrasound estimating the fetal weight to be 4100 grams. Her two previous pregnancies, also complicated by gestational diabetes, resulted in vaginal deliveries of 8- and 9-pound infants, who are both alive and without problems. She is admitted to labor and delivery. Oxytocin is added for labor augmentation. Upon rupture of membranes, meconium is present. Cervical change continues but is protracted, changing about 1 cm every 2 hours until she finally reaches 10 cm. She pushes for 2 hours, and after the head is delivered it retracts slightly back toward the vagina.

1. Which of the following should *not* be done at this time?
   A. Indicate to those present that a shoulder dystocia is present.
   B. Call for assistance.
   C. Suction meconium from the nasopharynx.
   D. Perform McRoberts' maneuver.
   E. Ask a nurse to apply suprapubic pressure.
2. Which of the following puts the fetus at greatest risk of shoulder dystocia?
   A. Multiparity
   B. Well-controlled maternal gestational diabetes
   C. Fetal macrosomia
   D. Protracted active phase
   E. Prior shoulder dystocia
3. Which of the following is the most common sequelae of a shoulder dystocia that can give long-term impairment?
   A. Klumpke paralysis
   B. Erb-Duchenne paralysis
   C. Fractured clavicle
   D. Fractured humerus

## COMMENT

**Risk factors for shoulder dystocia** • Recognition of the risk factors for a shoulder dystocia is the first step in minimizing complications. The most common risk factor is macrosomia. An estimated fetal weight greater than 4000 g increases risk about 10-fold (to 3% to 4%). If fetal weight is greater than 4500 g, risk is increased about 20-fold (about 8%). Gestational diabetes not only increases the likelihood of macrosomia, but also changes the weight distribution of a fetus. Increased mass around the chest and shoulders increases incidence of dystocia even if diabetes is well controlled and macrosomia is not present.

If the course of active labor is protracted (a slow rate of cervical change), the risk of malpresentation, cesarean section, and shoulder dystocia is increased. Other factors associated with shoulder dystocia are maternal obesity, previous birth of an infant over 4000 g, previous shoulder dystocia, and instrumental midpelvic delivery.

**Initial maneuvers to relieve shoulder dystocia** • Early recognition of a shoulder dystocia allows a rapid response and maximizes the time allowed to complete the delivery. All medical personnel present should be informed that a dystocia is present, and if enough assistants are not present, they should be called. The patient should be placed in McRoberts' position, in which the hips are hyperflexed and knees brought up to the shoulders. This opens the maternal pelvis. If delivery is not accomplished, applying pressure immediately above the symphysis pubis can dislodge the fetal shoulder from its trapped position. These two maneuvers will resolve 90% of shoulder dystocias.

Although suction with a DeLee catheter is usually performed after delivery of the fetal head in the presence of meconium, this step is skipped with shoulder dystocia. The momentum of delivery is not interrupted, since taking time to suction will allow further retraction of the head.

**Sequelae of shoulder dystocia** • The perinatal death rate from shoulder dystocia ranges from 19 to 289 per 1000. Erb-Duchenne palsy, or paralysis of the upper arm due to damage of C5-C6 in the brachial plexus, may result from excess traction on the fetal head. It occurs in 9% to 10% of cases. Klumpke palsy, paralysis of the lower arm and hand, results from brachial plexus trauma in C8-T1, and occurs in 2% to 3% of cases. About 15% of all palsies will have permanent disabilities. A fractured clavicle from suprapubic pressure or fractured humerus during attempted delivery of the posterior arm occur about 20% of the time, but almost never lead to long-term deficits.

**Answers** • 1-C 2-C 3-B

## CASE PRESENTATION

A 33-year-old woman presents to your office with the complaint of continued vaginal discharge. The onset of the discharge was approximately 6 days ago and is not resolving. She describes the discharge as thin, gray, and malodorous. She denies irregular vaginal bleeding. She is sexually active with her partner of 10 years. They do not use condoms. She denies any history of sexually transmitted diseases. She reports douching 1 week prior to the office visit.

1. Which of the following is the most likely diagnosis?
   A. Cervical dysplasia
   B. Vaginal candidiasis
   C. Bacterial vaginosis
   D. *Chlamydia* cervicitis
   E. None of the above
2. Which of the following would most likely aid you the most in your diagnosis?
   A. Complete blood count with differential
   B. Wet prep
   C. Culture for gonorrhea and *Chlamydia* infection
   D. Pap smear
   E. None of the above
3. Which of the following would you expect to see to help confirm your diagnosis?
   A. Hyphae
   B. Multiple white blood cells
   C. Cue cells
   D. Normal squamous epithelial cells
   E. None of the above
4. You decide to check the vaginal pH to aid in your diagnosis. You expect it to be:
   A. 1.5 to 2.4
   B. 2.5 to 3.4
   C. 3.5 to 4.4
   D. Greater than 4.5
   E. None of the above
5. What would you use for first-line therapy?
   A. Fluconazole
   B. Metronidazole
   C. Cryotherapy
   D. Azithromycin
   E. None of the above

## COMMENT

**Signs and symptoms of bacterial vaginosis** • This patient presents with the classic signs and symptoms of bacterial vaginosis. Bacterial vaginosis is usually accompanied by the complaint of a thin, gray vaginal discharge. The discharge is described as having a "fishy" odor. The odor is a result of amine by-products produced by anaerobic bacteria. Bacterial vaginosis is thought to occur when the normal flora of the vagina, *Lactobacillus*, is eradicated and replaced by multiple bacterial species. Douching may cause this eradication. Candidiasis characteristically is associated with a thick, white, "cottage cheese" discharge and vulvar or vaginal pruritus. No odor is often noted. *Chlamydia trachomatis,* a sexually transmitted disease, is associated with a yellow, mucopurulent discharge and no itching. This would further narrow the differential diagnosis because this patient is in a monogamous relationship. Cervical dysplasia is typically not associated with a characteristic discharge, but bleeding due to ulceration or friability of the cervix may occur.

**Diagnostic test** • A wet prep is a beneficial diagnostic tool when evaluating vaginal discharge. The characteristic finding of bacterial vaginosis is the presence of clue cells. *Clue cells* are squamous epithelial cells with adherent bacteria. Due to the adherent bacteria, the squamous cells have irregular, obscured borders rather than their original smooth, demarcated borders. A complete blood count with differential and cultures for *Chlamydia* would be helpful to rule out sexually transmitted disease or pelvic inflammatory disease. A Pap smear would screen for cervical dysplasia.

**Wet prep findings** • As stated previously, the finding associated with bacterial vaginosis is characteristic clue cells. Hyphae or pseudohyphae would be seen in the presence of candidiasis. Multiple white blood cells indicate inflammation due to cervicitis or pelvic inflammatory disease.

**pH of vagina** • The normal pH of the vagina is in the range of 3.8 to 4.2. This acidic environment, due to the production of lactic acid by the *Lactobacilli* species, maintains the normal vaginal flora. pH paper can be placed on the wall of the vagina to aid in the diagnosis of vaginal discharge. The vaginal pH associated with bacterial vaginosis is greater than 4.5. This alkalinization is caused by an overgrowth of Gram-negative and Gram-positive anaerobes, which have eradicated the stabilizing *Lactobacilli* of the vagina. Alkalinization has been attributed to frequent intercourse and douching.

**Treatment of bacterial vaginosis** • Metronidazole and clindamycin are the two antimicrobial agents approved for the treatment of bacterial vaginosis. Fluconazole is an antifungal used for the treatment of vaginal candidiasis. *Chlamydia* infection may be treated with azithromycin, a macrolide antibiotic. Cryotherapy is an option for the eradication of cervical dysplasia.

**Answers** • 1-C 2-B 3-C 4-C 5-B

## CASE PRESENTATION

A 26-year-old G2P1 at 31 1/7 weeks' gestation presents complaining of uterine contractions every 5 minutes for the last 3 to 4 hours. She has had a clear, slightly blood-tinged discharge for the last 4 days. Her pregnancy has thus far been uncomplicated, but her last pregnancy resulted in a preterm birth at 33 weeks. On physical exam, she is afebrile with normal blood pressure. The abdomen is nontender except with contractions, which are palpable and firm.

1. Which of the following tests or therapies should be avoided at this time?
   A. Urine and cervical cultures
   B. External monitoring of fetal heart rate and tocometer
   C. Digital cervical exam
   D. Intravenous hydration
   E. Sterile speculum exam
2. A sterile speculum exam is performed, which shows a discharge but no evidence of rupture of membranes. By digital exam, the cervix is 3 cm dilated, 50% effaced, and the fetus is in a high station. The fetal heart tone is in the 130s, with several accelerations and excellent variability. After IV hydration, contractions continue every 5 minutes. The best management at this time would be:
   A. Continue hydration
   B. Initiate tocolysis with magnesium sulfate
   C. Administer antibiotics for group B streptococcus (GBS) coverage
   D. Administer betamethasone
   E. All of the above
3. Which of the following places a pregnancy at the greatest risk of preterm birth?
   A. Twin gestation
   B. Polyhydramnios
   C. Multiparity
   D. Septate uterus
   E. History of cervical cone biopsy
4. Which of the following is not a side effect of tocolysis with magnesium sulfate or indomethacin?
   A. Maternal pulmonary edema
   B. Decreased maternal reflexes
   C. Fever
   D. Constriction of the fetal ductus arteriosus
   E. Fetal oligohydramnios
5. Which of the following is true about preterm labor?
   A. Premature birth accounts for about 10% of the perinatal morbidity and mortality.
   B. Early diagnosis and treatment of preterm labor can significantly reduce the preterm birth rate.
   C. The overall incidence of preterm birth is 1% to 2%.
   D. Idiopathic preterm labor accounts for about one-third of preterm births.
   E. Weight at birth is a better predictor of neonatal outcome than gestational age.

**Answers** • 1-C 2-E 3-A 4-C 5-D

## COMMENT

**Evaluation of preterm complaints** • This patient has complaints consistent with preterm labor. The definition of preterm labor is regular uterine contractions with resulting cervical change occurring before 37 weeks' gestation. Because this patient reports leaking of fluid, a speculum exam should be done first to exclude rupture of the membranes (ROM). A cervical check should only be done if this is negative, since a check in the presence of ROM increases the risk of chorioamnionitis. A urinalysis, urine culture, and cervical swab for PCR analysis of gonorrhea and *Chlamydia* infection should be collected since a urinary tract infection or cervicitis can initiate preterm labor. Fetal well-being should be tested with a heart rate tracing. Tocometer tracing helps establish contraction frequency. Dehydration leads to increased antidiuretic hormone (ADH), which has homology with oxytocin and is capable of causing uterine contractions. Fluid administration corrects dehydration and may abate the contractions.

**Management of preterm labor** • Once the diagnosis of preterm labor is made, an attempt at tocolysis is made if fetal status is reassuring. The tocolytic most commonly used is magnesium sulfate. The immediate goal of tocolysis is to delay delivery for at least 24 to 48 hours so that steroids can be administered (betamethasone, two doses of 12 mg 24 hours apart) to decrease neonatal morbidities. Antibiotics to cover group B streptococcus are appropriate in cases of threatened preterm delivery, since these neonates are especially susceptible to GBS sepsis.

**Conditions associated with preterm labor** • Identification of risk factors for preterm labor can lead to early intervention and early therapy. Twin gestation places a patient and fetus at the highest risk: Almost 50% of patients deliver before 37 weeks. Any condition that leads to overdistension of the uterus, such as twin gestation or polyhydramnios, increases the incidence of uterine activity and preterm labor. Uterine anomalies are associated with early and abnormal contraction patterns. These include septate uterus, didelphic uterus, and fibroids. Cervical incompetence, defined as painless cervical dilatation, is associated with preterm birth. This is most often idiopathic, but patients with a history of cervical surgery, including conization or surgical dilation, are at increased risk. Patients with a history of preterm birth are at risk for recurrence, but multiparity alone is not a risk factor.

**Complications of treatment of preterm labor** • Magnesium is associated with development of pulmonary edema and decreased peripheral muscle reflexes. Indomethacin, an inhibitor of prostaglandin production and potent tocolytic, can also cause constriction of the fetal ductus arteriosus and oligohydramnios. These effects are reversible if indomethacin is discontinued, so it is generally used for only 48-hour courses. Although patients being treated for preterm labor may develop fever, it should be seen as a sign of chorioamnionitis, not attributed to side effects of therapy. Delivery in these patients should be augmented to minimize risk of neonatal sepsis.

**Preterm labor statistics** • Preterm births account for more than 50% of all neonatal morbidity and mortality. Despite an increased understanding of the pathophysiology of preterm labor, the morbidity and mortality from this condition over the last 50 years has not been decreased despite earlier diagnosis and tocolytics that can abate uterine contractions. Premature birth complicates about 10% of all pregnancies. Approximately one-third of these are due to fetal or maternal complications (hypertensive disorders, placental accidents, congenital abnormalities), about one-third are due to preterm premature rupture of membranes (PPROM), and about one-third are due to "idiopathic" preterm labor. The most important predictor of neonatal outcome, all other factors being equal, is gestational age at delivery. Given the same gestational age, however, a larger infant will have a better prognosis.

## CASE PRESENTATION

A 27-year-old patient complains of 8 months of dysmenorrhea uncontrolled by oral contraceptives and nonsteroidal anti-inflammatory agents (NSAIDs). The pain is often present between periods. She has had a cesarean section and surgery for a ruptured appendix. The pain has caused her to miss about 4 days of work each month. Tylenol does not help, but narcotics given to her from an emergency room visit work relatively well. A physical exam shows tenderness throughout the lower pelvis, a normal-sized uterus, and normal ovaries. However, the uterus is not very mobile.

1. Of the following, the best next step would be to:
   - A. Order a pelvic CT
   - B. Prescribe narcotics for monthly use during menses
   - C. Obtain a psychiatry consult
   - D. Perform diagnostic laparoscopy
   - E. Perform a hysterectomy
2. The patient is taken to surgery, where moderate pelvic adhesions are seen. Also noted are multiple charcoal-colored circular spots about 1 to 2 mm, located on the ovary and in the cul-de-sac. Which of the following is most appropriate management?
   - A. Destruction of the lesions and postoperative oral contraceptives
   - B. Hysterectomy with bilateral salpingo-oophorectomy
   - C. No intraoperative procedures, with postoperative oral contraceptives
   - D. No intraoperative procedures, with postoperative gonadotropin-releasing hormone (GnRH) agonist therapy
3. The same patient presents at age 47. She has enjoyed many pain-free years after diagnosis and treatment of endometriosis, but now her dysmenorrhea has returned. There is no pain between menses. Her menses are heavier than usual, with duration increasing to 6 days (from 3) and flow increasing to 9 pads per day (from 4 to 5) over the last year. She reports pressure symptoms with menses. NSAIDs and acetaminophen are ineffective. She is now divorced and is not sexually active. Exam shows a 12-week-size uterus with a boggy consistency that is tender to palpation. The adnexa feel normal. What is the most appropriate next step?
   - A. Pelvic ultrasound
   - B. Hysterectomy with bilateral salpingo-oophorectomy
   - C. Endometrial biopsy
   - D. Diagnostic laparoscopy
   - E. Antibiotics for endometritis
4. An endometrial biopsy is performed, showing secretory endometrium without hyperplasia, carcinoma, or endometritis. An ultrasound is ordered, showing an enlarged uterus without fibroids. The adnexa are normal. Given the symptoms described above, the most likely diagnosis is:
   - A. Intracavitary fibroids
   - B. Adenomyosis
   - C. Recurrent endometriosis
   - D. Diverticulitis
   - E. Pelvic adhesive disease

## COMMENT

**Chronic pelvic pain** • This patient has a diagnosis of chronic pelvic pain, since it has been present for more than 6 months and is causing a significant disruption in her ability to manage her life. Given her surgical history, pelvic adhesive disease is a strong possibility. However, adhesion formation is variable from patient to patient. To make a diagnosis and select appropriate therapy, a diagnostic laparoscopy is indicated, since an adequate trial of medical management has failed. Laparoscopy may be therapeutic as well if adhesions or endometriotic implants are excised and/or destroyed at the time of surgery. 75% of patients will get relief from laparoscopy regardless of pathology or diagnosis, but in 50% of these patients, pain will recur.

Chronic narcotic use is only acceptable in incurable disease states. Some physicians would order an ultrasound even with a normal exam, looking for an ovarian cyst or uterine pathology, but a CT scan is less accurate. A hysterectomy is not indicated until other therapeutic alternatives with less morbidity are attempted. A psychiatric component such as a history of sexual abuse is common with chronic pelvic pain. A thorough history should be taken, but a psychiatric consult is only useful if the patient reports suicidal ideation or other signs of clinical depression.

**Diagnosis and treatment of endometriosis** • Endometriosis classically has the appearance of "powder-burn lesions" attached to the peritoneum. These may be superficially attached or more invasive and fixed. The most common locations of endometriosis are on the ovary and in the cul-de-sac, consistent with one proposed mechanism of endometriosis, backflow of endometrial tissue through the fallopian tubes. Endometriosis is often accompanied by pelvic adhesions, as a result of repeated turnover of damaged peritoneal surfaces from endometriotic implant bleeding. Treatment consists of ablation or excision of the implants at the time of surgery and postoperative ovulation suppression, either with oral contraceptives, medroxyprogesterone acetate, or short-term GnRH analogs. Recurrence is common, and a hysterectomy is appropriate in the patient who is refractory to therapy and no longer wishes to preserve fertility. However, hysterectomy should not be done as a first-line treatment, since success rates with conservative treatment are good and hysterectomy has higher operative morbidity and longer recovery time.

**Endometrial biopsy in perimenopausal bleeding** • Any patient over the age of 40 (some authorities recommend 35) with an increase in menses, either by report of menorrhagia or by onset of intermenstrual bleeding, should have an endometrial biopsy to exclude hyperplasia or malignancy. A pelvic ultrasound is a good idea in a patient whose exam is difficult to interpret, in whom endometrial biopsy is not possible, or in whom it is necessary to rule out an adnexal mass. Laparoscopy and hysterectomy are not appropriate until malignancy is excluded with biopsy. This patient does not have risk factors for endometritis (i.e., unprotected intercourse, recent uterine instrumentation, or being postpartum), so antibiotics are not indicated unless suggested on biopsy result.

**Adenomyosis** • Although all of the diagnoses listed are possibilities, adenomyosis is the most likely choice. Adenomyosis results from ectopic implants of endometrial tissue in the myometrium. The uterus is diffusely enlarged and has a boggy consistency. Like endometriosis, the diagnosis can be suspected on history and physical, but only confirmed pathologically. Hysterectomy is indicated and curative.

**Answers** • 1-D 2-A 3-C 4-B

## CASE PRESENTATION

A 40-year-old African American G2P2 woman presents to your office complaining of increasing duration of menses as well as increasing pain and cramping. Menarche occurred at age 13. Her menses did occur every 28 days and would last 5 days in duration. She now reports menses 12 days in length with large clots. She changes a soaked sanitary napkin every 2 hours. She denies syncope but reports increased lethargy. She has no significant past medical history. She takes no medications. Her physical exam reveals blood pressure 126/76, pulse 88, weight 152 lb, height 5 feet 7 inches. Heart and lung exams are within normal limits. Abdomen is soft, nontender, slightly distended, no rebound or guarding, no organomegaly. Pelvic exam reveals normal vagina, no discharge or active bleeding, cervix without lesions, uterus enlarged, irregular in shape, 14 weeks' size, mobile and nontender. No adnexal masses are appreciated. Urine βhCG is negative. Hemoglobin is 9.2 mg/dL. She smokes one pack of cigarettes per day. An endometrial biopsy was performed, which revealed benign proliferative endometrium.

1. The correct medical terminology for her symptom of increased menstruation is:
   A. Dysmenorrhea
   B. Metrorrhagia
   C. Menorrhagia
   D. Menometrorrhagia
   E. None of the above
2. After performing the history and physical, your most likely diagnosis is:
   A. Cervical carcinoma
   B. Endometrial carcinoma
   C. Endometrial polyp
   D. Leiomyomata
   E. None of the above
3. Which of the following is a possible treatment option for this patient?
   A. Total abdominal hysterectomy
   B. Laparoscopically assisted vaginal hysterectomy
   C. Uterine artery embolization
   D. All of the above
   E. None of the above
4. The patient declines any invasive procedures and would like to begin with medical management. Which of the following are treatment options?
   A. IM gonadotropin-releasing hormone (GnRH) agonist
   B. Cyclical oral progesterone
   C. IM medroxyprogesterone
   D. All of the above
   E. None of the above
5. The patient is unsure regarding future pregnancies. The best surgical management for her would be:
   A. Supracervical hysterectomy
   B. Myomectomy
   C. Endometrial ablation by roller ball
   D. Endometrial ablation by thermal balloon
   E. None of the above

## COMMENT

**Definition of menorrhagia** • Menorrhagia is defined as menses greater than 8 days in length or loss of menstrual blood exceeding 80 mL. Because this patient has menses 12 days in duration, changes a pad every 2 hours, and is anemic, her symptoms are defined as menorrhagia. Dysmenorrhea simply indicates painful menses. Metrorrhagia indicates intermenstrual bleeding or irregularly timed bleeding. Menometrorrhagia describes menses with both menorrhagia and metrorrhagia symptomatology.

**Etiology of menorrhagia** • With menorrhagia and a 12-week-size irregularly shaped uterus, the most likely working diagnosis would be leiomyomata, commonly known as fibroids. Uterine leiomyomata are benign smooth muscle tumors. They may be subserosal, intramural, or submucosal in location. Leiomyomata appear to be more common in African American women. They often are asymptomatic and found solely upon examination. Symptoms produced by fibroids may include irregular menstrual bleeding, pelvic pain and pressure, dysmenorrhea, and dyspareunia. Endometrial polyps usually present with metrorrhagia or mild irregular spotting. Diagnosis and treatment include hysteroscopy with dilatation and curettage. Endometrial carcinoma is not likely, since the endometrial biopsy was negative. Carcinoma of the uterus is most often seen in postmenopausal women or women with excess of estrogen. This patient takes no unopposed estrogen and is not overweight to cause aromatization. Cervical carcinoma is highly unlikely because this patient denies postcoital bleeding, has had normal annual exams, and her cervix is without lesions.

**Surgical treatment options** • Leiomyomata may be treated with both surgical and medical management. Abdominal hysterectomy and laparoscopically assisted vaginal hysterectomy are both certainly options for surgical management. As the uterus approaches 14 weeks' size, some surgeons prefer to proceed with abdominal surgery rather than the vaginal route. Uterine artery embolization is becoming a more common treatment for symptomatic fibroid uteri. Using a polyvinyl gel, the uterine artery is partially occluded via catheterization. This occlusion causes infarct of the fibroids, resulting in shrinkage of the fibroids and decreased symptoms.

**Medical treatment options** • All of the choices listed are appropriate medical management for fibroids with menorrhagia. Cyclic progesterone for 12 days of the cycle, inducing a withdrawal bleed, may produce a normal menses. IM medroxyprogesterone (Depo-Provera) often can decrease bleeding by inducing a state of amenorrhea. GnRH agonists given in one large IM dose place the patient in a state of temporary menopause, ceasing menstruation. GnRH agonist therapy decreases the size of uterine fibroids due to lack of estrogen stimulation. Menopausal symptoms such as hot flashes and mood swings may be experienced. GnRH agonist use should be limited to 3 months because side effects such as osteoporosis can occur. GnRH agonist therapy is the most costly of the choices.

**Preserving fertility** • Of the choices listed, myomectomy (surgical removal of leiomyomas) is the only procedure that would preserve fertility. Patients need to be aware that myomas may have a 50% recurrence rate within 5 years of myomectomy, which may lead to future surgeries. Myomas cause infertility due to distortion of the uterine cavity or by tubal occlusion. Endometrial ablation by either method destroys the endometrium, making pregnancy unlikely. Supracervical hysterectomy would not be an option because the uterus is surgically removed with preservation of the cervix.

**Answers** • 1-C 2-D 3-D 4-D 5-B

## CASE PRESENTATION

A 32-year-old G3P2 at 31 2/7 weeks presents reporting a gush of clear fluid per vagina after standing up early that day. She has not felt any contractions, and the baby is moving well. Her pregnancy has been uncomplicated thus far, except for a history of deliveries "about a month early." Her cervix has been checked routinely in clinic because of this history, and has always been closed. She is afebrile, with a pulse of 94. The uterus is nontender, and the fetal heart rate tracing shows excellent variability and three 15-beat accelerations with no decelerations. The tocometer does not show any contractions.

1. Which of the following is not part of the triad of tests for rupture of the membranes?
   - A. Pooling of fluid in the vaginal vault
   - B. Ferning pattern on dry slide preparation
   - C. Amniotic fluid index less than 5 cm
   - D. Basic pH of vaginal secretions
2. Which of the following is not a sign of chorioamnionitis?
   - A. Increased fetal movement
   - B. Uterine tenderness
   - C. Maternal tachycardia
   - D. Fetal tachycardia
   - E. Fever
3. If clinical chorioamnionitis is not present with preterm premature rupture of the membranes (PPROM), betamethasone should be given:
   - A. To all patients who are preterm (less than 37 weeks)
   - B. Only to patients less than 34 weeks
   - C. Only to patients less than 32 weeks
   - D. Only to patients less than 28 weeks
   - E. To no patients with PPROM
4. Benefits of betamethasone include:
   - A. Acceleration of fetal lung maturity
   - B. Decreased incidence of necrotizing enterocolitis
   - C. Decreased incidence of intraventricular hemorrhage
   - D. Decreased incidence of cerebral palsy
   - E. A, B, and C
5. Microorganisms targeted with administration of antibiotics to PPROM patients include:
   - A. Gram-positive cocci
   - B. Gram-negative bacilli
   - C. Anaerobes
   - D. Atypical bacteria
   - E. All of the above

## COMMENT

**Diagnosis of rupture of the membranes** • The classic triad of rupture of the membranes (ROM) is pooling of amniotic fluid in the vaginal vault, basic pH of fluid in the vault, and a ferning pattern seen under the microscope, as estrogen-complexed salt crystallizes on a dry slide. The most specific of these is pooling of fluid. A urinary tract infection with *Proteus* species or blood in the vagina can lead to a false positive alkaline test. The high estrogen content in cervical mucous can sometimes show a ferning pattern. However, when all three are present, the diagnosis is established. Oligohydramnios, defined as an amniotic fluid index of less than 5 cm, is often seen after rupture of membranes, but patients with ROM may have more residual fluid than this, and there are other causes of oligohydramnios. The amniotic fluid index may be used to suspect ROM if the diagnosis is unclear, but the other three tests are more specific to ROM.

**Signs of chorioamnionitis** • Chorioamnionitis results from the ascent of bacterial flora of the vagina and resulting infection of the chorion and amnion surrounding the fetus. This most often occurs after prolonged rupture of membranes, either preterm or during term labor. It can occur before the rupture of membranes, however, and is a common cause of preterm labor. The classic triad of chorioamnionitis is maternal tachycardia, fetal tachycardia, and uterine tenderness. Other common signs are fever, increased uterine activity, and leukocytosis. The infection surrounding the fetus may result in *decreased* fetal movement and decreased variability on a fetal heart rate tracing.

**Gestational age for steroid administration in PPROM patients** • The benefit of steroids to preterm infants must be balanced with the risk of perpetuating or facilitating an infection, most specifically chorioamnionitis. In patients with intact membranes and the threat of early delivery, steroids are given until 34 weeks' gestation. In patients with PROM, however, steroids are generally not given after 32 weeks' gestation, since the risk/benefit ratio is different: The risk of developing chorioamnionitis is higher when PROM is present, and steroids would exacerbate morbidity from this condition. Chorioamnionitis may be suggested by significant uterine contractions, fever, maternal or fetal tachycardia, or fundal tenderness.

**Benefits of betamethasone** • Betamethasone therapy has been shown to accelerate maturation of type II pneumocytes and increased production of surfactant, decreasing the incidence of neonatal respiratory distress. It also decreases the incidence of necrotizing enterocolitis and intraventricular hemorrhage, common significant complications of prematurity. The incidence of cerebral palsy is not significantly decreased by betamethasone administration.

**Antibiotics for PPROM** • Antimicrobial therapy for PPROM has two goals: prolonging latency (the time from rupture of membranes to delivery) and minimizing neonatal group B streptococcal (GBS) infection. GBS is a Gram-positive cocci. The organisms that would contribute to chorioamnionitis and decrease latency are those that normally exist in the vagina or may initiate infection, and include Gram-negative bacilli, anaerobes, and atypical organisms. Many regimens may cover all of these, but the best studies showing prolonged latency used ampicillin (which covers GBS and anaerobes well, and has fairly good Gram-negative coverage) and azithromycin (for atypical coverage such as *Chlamydia* and *Ureaplasma* species). Current recommendations are a 7-day course of ampicillin (or amoxicillin for oral dosing) and azithromycin.

**Answers** • 1-C 2-A 3-C 4-E 5-E

## CASE PRESENTATION

A 47-year-old African American woman presents with the complaint of a heavy period, lasting for 12 days, requiring the use of 6 to 9 pads per day. It is the first period she has had in the last 4 months. Her menses have been less frequent over the last 2 years, approximately once every 3 months, accompanied by hot flashes and increased irritability. She denies weight loss or change in appetite. An abdominal and pelvic exam is negative, with apparently normal-size uterus and adnexa, though it is limited by her moderate obesity

1. What is the most appropriate next step?
   A. Endometrial biopsy
   B. Pelvic ultrasound
   C. Pelvic CT scan
   D. Hormonal therapy
   E. Reassurance that the bleeding is normal and reexamine in 3 months
2. The endometrial biopsy shows simple hyperplasia. Which of the following is the most appropriate therapy?
   A. Expectant management with repeat endometrial biopsy in 3 months
   B. Continuous conjugated estrogens 0.625 mg and cyclic medroxyprogesterone acetate 10 mg
   C. Cyclic medroxyprogesterone acetate 10 mg
   D. Simple hysterectomy with bilateral salpingo-oophorectomy
   E. Radical hysterectomy with bilateral salpingo-oophorectomy and lymph node sampling
3. A similar patient has a biopsy return complex hyperplasia with atypia. A dilation and curettage is performed, which shows adenocarcinoma, grade 2, with a negative endocervical curettage. The next appropriate step is:
   A. Continue cyclic progesterone with resampling in 3 months
   B. Simple vaginal hysterectomy with bilateral salpingo-oophorectomy
   C. Referral to a gynecologic oncologist for abdominal hysterectomy with salpingo-oophorectomy and possible lymph node dissection
   D. Radical hysterectomy with salpingo-oophorectomy
   E. External beam radiation
4. Which of the following is true about endometrial adenocarcinoma?
   A. Factors associated with unopposed estrogen increase a patient's risk.
   B. It is clinically staged.
   C. It is the third most common gynecologic malignancy in the United States.
   D. The endometrial biopsy is an effective screening test.
   E. Multiparity is a risk factor for development.

## COMMENT

**Evaluation of postmenopausal bleeding** • In any woman older than 40 (some recommend 35) with increased vaginal bleeding in the form of heaviness (menorrhagia) or irregularity (metrorrhagia), it is important to exclude the presence of endometrial hyperplasia or adenocarcinoma. This condition may exist despite a normal exam, ultrasound, or CT scan. Cyclic hormonal therapy in the form of oral contraceptive pills or a cyclic progestational agent will more than likely regulate her bleeding, but a malignancy must first be excluded.

**Treatment of simple hyperplasia** • There are four classes of endometrial hyperplasia: simple hyperplasia, complex hyperplasia, simple hyperplasia with atypia, and complex hyperplasia with atypia. The risk of malignancy goes up with each class (approximately 1%, 3%, 8%, and 25%, respectively). Simple hyperplasia may be treated with a cyclic progestational agent. One would not want to add estrogen to an estrogen-dependent process such as endometrial hyperplasia. A simple hysterectomy is an option in all patients with hyperplasia, but in *simple* hyperplasia the cure rate is so high and the risk of cancer is so low that the morbidity from total abdominal hysterectomy and bilateral salpingo-oophorectomy (TAHBSO) is unnecessary. All conservatively managed patients require resampling of the endometrial cavity 3 months after hormonal therapy begins. Resolution of hyperplasia allows continuation of conservative management, whereas persistence or progression to a more atypical class (or carcinoma) warrants surgical treatment.

**Treatment of endometrial adenocarcinoma** • The standard treatment of endometrial cancer is TAHBSO regardless of the patient's age. For low-grade stage I disease this affords a greater than 90% cure rate. Whether or not to perform lymph node dissection for low-grade early-stage disease is controversial and evolving. Therefore, referral to a gynecologic oncologist who is apprised of the most recent literature and is trained to perform lymph node dissection is most appropriate. A lymphadenectomy would definitely be indicated for high-grade or high-stage lesions.

Removal of the parametria (broad, cardinal, and uterosacral ligaments), as accomplished by a radical hysterectomy, is usually unnecessary for endometrial cancer and carries excess morbidity. This is the preferred operation for cervical cancer. External beam radiation is reserved for cases of recurrence, cases with lymph node involvement or deep myometrial invasion, and preoperatively for bulky tumors.

**Facts about endometrial adenocarcinoma** • Most endometrial adenocarcinomas are examples of a hormonally dependent carcinoma. Stages of development can be identified, from hyperplasia to atypical hyperplasia to carcinoma. Patients at risk for developing this disease are those with chronic unopposed estrogenic stimulation, such as chronic anovulation. Exogenous progesterone should be given to these patients. Staging for endometrial cancer is surgical, not clinical as it is for cervical cancer. In the United States, uterine cancer is the most common gynecologic malignancy (about 35,000 cases per year), followed by ovarian cancer (about 25,000 cases per year), and finally cervical cancer (15,000 cases per year). However, because of the lack of health care and preventive care programs in underdeveloped countries, cervical cancer remains the most common gynecologic cancer worldwide. Unlike for cervical cancer, there is no reliable screening test for endometrial cancer. The endometrial biopsy is diagnostic. Most patients will present with abnormal uterine bleeding.

**Answers** • 1-A 2-C 3-C 4-A

## CASE PRESENTATION

A 28-year-old G3P2 with a 39 4/7 weeks' intrauterine pregnancy presents with the complaint of bright red blood noted on her underwear. She denies contractions, loss of fluid, or abdominal pain. She reports good fetal movement. Her past obstetrical history is significant for two cesarean sections for arrest of dilatation. She has no significant past medical history. She denies tobacco, alcohol, or any recreational drug use. Her vitals upon presentation include blood pressure 90/50, temperature 98.8°F, pulse 112, respirations 22. Her abdominal exam is soft and nontender. Fetal heart tones are in the 170s with fair beat to beat variability. No decelerations are identified. Tocometer shows occasional irregular contractions.

1. Which of the following is the most likely diagnosis?
   - A. Latent labor
   - B. Abruptio placenta
   - C. Placenta previa
   - D. Chorioamnionitis
   - E. None of the above
2. Which of the following actions should be performed next?
   - A. Digital cervical examination
   - B. Amniocentesis
   - C. Urine drug screen
   - D. Fetal ultrasound
   - E. All of the above
3. Your suspicion is confirmed. The next step in the management of this patient is:
   - A. Begin oxytocin for augmentation of labor
   - B. Perform biophysical profile and, if it's reassuring, have patient return in 1 week
   - C. Proceed with cesarean section
   - D. Begin IV antibiotics
   - E. None of the above
4. Which of the following risks must you discuss with this patient prior to initiation of your management?
   - A. Possible uterine rupture when beginning oxytocin
   - B. Possible placenta accreta necessitating hysterectomy
   - C. Possible risk of hemorrhage at home while on bed rest
   - D. Possible sepsis
   - E. None of the above

## COMMENT

**Third trimester bleeding** • Presentation of bright red vaginal bleeding should bring several different possibilities to mind. Bleeding may be caused by a simple, straightforward reason such as bleeding from the cervix due to recent intercourse, inflammation due to infection, or cervical change due to labor. More worrisome causes must also be considered. Abruption should be considered but is often accompanied by abdominal pain and tetanic contractions. Additionally, this patient has no risk factors for abruption such as trauma, hypertension, or cocaine use. With painless vaginal bleeding, placenta previa should be suspected. Placenta previa can quickly become an emergent situation if bleeding ensues. Chorioamnionitis is unlikely in this patient because there is no evidence of maternal fever or abdominal tenderness. Chorioamnionitis is usually not accompanied by bleeding.

**Contraindications for placenta previa** • Because placenta previa is the most likely diagnosis, a digital cervical exam is contraindicated. Identifying the location of the placenta is imperative. With increasing clarity of ultrasound, the placenta can usually be identified using the abdominal, transvaginal, or transperineal approach. Amniocentesis is usually performed to diagnose intrauterine infection and identify chromosomal abnormalities. Information from an amniocentesis would not be helpful regarding this patient. A urine drug screen is helpful to rule out substance abuse. This would be more beneficial if abruptio placenta was highly suspected.

**Treatment of placenta previa** • With active bleeding and evidence of placenta previa in a term pregnancy, delivery by cesarean section is indicated. Vaginal delivery or augmentation of labor is contraindicated in this patient. Preterm pregnancies with minimal bleeding and contractions may be offered a trial of tocolysis with magnesium sulfate. With minimal bleeding and no contractions, bed rest in the hospital setting would be an option. Discharging a patient home would not be the standard of care, as bleeding can become catastrophic within seconds. Any patient with known previa should have typed and cross-matched blood immediately available.

**Risk factors associated with placenta previa** • Any patient with a previous cesarean section and currently confirmed previa should be counseled regarding her risk of placenta accreta. Placenta accreta is defined as invasion of placental tissue into the myometrium of the uterus. The risk of placenta accreta in a patient with a previa and prior cesarean section is approximately 10% to 20%. This risk increases with each cesarean section performed. By the time a women has her fourth cesarean section, the risk for accreta may be as high as 65%. At the time of cesarean section the placenta is unable to separate from the uterine wall, resulting in hemorrhage. The treatment for placenta accreta is hysterectomy. Because hysterectomy renders the patient infertile, this must be discussed with the patient prior to cesarean section.

**Answers** • 1-D 2-D 3-C 4-B

## CASE PRESENTATION

A 58-year-old white woman is noted to have an enlarged adnexa during her annual exam. On review of systems, she reports increased abdominal girth, heartburn, bloating, and decreased appetite. An ultrasound is ordered, showing a 12-cm right-sided mass with multiple septations, and significant ascites. A cancer antigen 125 (CA125) test is 789 (normal, <30).

1. Which of the following statements about ovarian cancer is true?
   A. A woman's lifetime risk of ovarian cancer is 1% to 2%.
   B. Most ovarian cancer patients have a BRCA1 or BRCA2 mutation.
   C. Ovarian cancer is the most common gynecologic cancer.
   D. CA125 levels should be obtained yearly in high-risk patients.
   E. Most cases are advanced at diagnosis because of aggressive hematologic spread.
2. The patient is referred to a gynecologic oncologist who performs total abdominal hysterectomy, bilateral salpingo-oophorectomy, omentectomy, and lymph node dissection. The ascitic fluid is sent for cytologic analysis. Which one of these statements about pathologic findings is true?
   A. The most likely pathologic type is mucinous cystadenocarcinoma.
   B. The contralateral ovary is more than 75% likely to be involved.
   C. Ovarian pathology is probably derived from the surface ovarian epithelium.
   D. Ovarian pathology is probably derived from a germ cell.
   E. Positive lymph nodes would give this patient stage IV diagnosis.
3. In a 35-year-old woman diagnosed with a stromal cell ovarian cancer, which of the following lab values would be the most likely to be elevated?
   A. Testosterone
   B. CA125
   C. Alpha-fetoprotein (AFP)
   D. Human chorionic gonadotropin (βhCG)
   E. Carcinoembryonic antigen (CEA)
4. Which one of the following is true about Krukenberg's tumors?
   A. They are ovarian malignancies that metastasize to distant sites.
   B. They most commonly result from metastatic colon cancer to the ovary.
   C. Patients with Krukenberg's tumors have a favorable prognosis after excision.
   D. If they contain metastatic thyroid tissue, they are called struma ovarii.
   E. The primary malignancy cannot be found in 10% of cases.

## COMMENT

**Ovarian cancer statistics** • A woman's lifetime risk of developing ovarian cancer is about 1.5%. It is the fifth most common cancer in women (about 25,000 cases per year), but third in mortality. Most women are in their 50s to 60s at diagnosis. The difficulty with ovarian cancer is that it is rarely symptomatic early in the disease process. About two-thirds of patients present with advanced disease, primarily by shedding of excrescences that grow on the surface of the ovary. These malignant cells break off and attach to bowel or omentum and are filtered by pelvic, periaortic, and subdiaphragmatic lymph nodes.

Only about 10% of all cases of ovarian cancer are thought to be due to an autosomal dominant pattern of inheritance; 90% of these are due to BRCA1 (70%) or BRCA2 (20%). Pelvic ultrasounds and CA125 tests have failed to show effectiveness as screening tools, even in high-risk patients, because of high false negative rates, which prevent diagnosis, and high false positive rates, which lead to unnecessary removal. Aside from prophylactic bilateral salpingo-oophorectomy, the only preventive measure known is long-term oral contraceptive use, which after 5 years can reduce lifetime risk of occurrence by 50%, even in BRCA-positive patients.

**Ovarian cancer pathology** • Ninety percent of ovarian cancers are of epithelial cell origin. The other two types, germ cell tumors and stromal cell tumors, are more common in younger women. Of the epithelial cell types, the most common is the serous cystadenocarcinoma. They are bilateral 30% of the time. Another common epithelial cancer, the mucinous cystadenocarcinoma, is less often bilateral (10% of the time) and is characteristically larger than the serous type. This may be associated with thick mucinous ascites, a condition called pseudomyxomatous peritonei. The third most common epithelial cell type is endometrioid, having features resembling the endometrial cavity. Clear cell carcinomas are the least common epithelial types. Lymph node involvement denotes stage IIIC ovarian cancer. Stage IV is diagnosed in the presence of distant metastasis.

**Ovarian cancer tumor markers** • Stromal cell neoplasms represent a higher percentage of neoplasms in middle-aged women. This type is often functional, or hormone producing. These are either from granulosa cells, which produce estrogens, or Sertoli-Leydig cells, which produce testosterone. The most common ovarian cancer type in women younger than 20 years is the germ cell tumor (easily remembered since this age population has the most germ cells). Four types are recognized: the dysgerminoma (most common), which is characteristically radiosensitive; the immature teratoma; the endodermal sinus tumor, which secretes AFP; and the embryonal cell carcinoma, which secretes AFP or βhCG or both.

**Krukenberg's tumors** • Krukenberg's tumors result from metastatic spread to the ovary from a distant primary. The most common primary site is gastric cancer (80%), showing characteristic signet ring cells on the pathologic specimen. Cancer may also metastasize to the ovary from the other ovary, breast, colon, and endometrium. In 10% of cases, the primary malignancy cannot be found despite a thorough workup. Prognosis in patients with Krukenberg's tumors is poor, with 5-year survival rates of about 5% to 10%. *Struma ovarii* is the term used for the rare variant of a dermoid cyst when benign functional thyroid tissue is present.

**Answers** • 1-A 2-C 3-A 4-E

## CASE PRESENTATION

A 41-year-old G3P1A1 Asian woman who is 16 weeks pregnant by a sure last menstrual period (LMP) presents to the emergency room complaining of vaginal bleeding for 2 days. She has had two doctor's visits this pregnancy. Because she was sure about her LMP, she has not yet had an ultrasound. She has used about 10 pads in the last 2 days. She has been nauseated for a week, the first nausea since early in the pregnancy. On exam her heart rate is 98, blood pressure is 135/88, and respiration rate 20. The uterus is to the level of the umbilicus, and nontender. A βhCG is drawn and returns 250,000 mIU/mL.

1. Which of the following should be done first to confirm the diagnosis?
   A. CT scan
   B. Abdominal ultrasound
   C. Prothrombin time/partial thromboplastin time (PT/PTT) and fibrin split products
   D. Dilation and curettage
   E. Cancer antigen 125 (CA125) test
2. What is the most likely genetic makeup in a molar pregnancy diagnosed by ultrasound?
   A. 69, XXX
   B. 69, XXY
   C. 46, XX
   D. 46, XY
   E. 45, XO
3. Which of the following differences between partial and complete moles are true?
   A. Partial moles are more likely to persist or become malignant or both.
   B. βhCG levels do not need to be monitored after evacuation of a partial mole.
   C. Complete moles may have small amounts of fetal tissue.
   D. Partial moles typically present earlier than complete moles.
   E. Medical complications such as preeclampsia, hyperthyroidism, and theca-lutein cysts are more common with complete moles.
4. Which of the following is not included in management of a molar pregnancy?
   A. Baseline βhCG levels
   B. Blood type and antibody screen
   C. Dilation and curettage
   D. Serum βhCG levels weekly until zero, then yearly for 5 years
   E. Reliable contraception
5. Which of the following is included in the management of persistent gestational trophoblastic disease (GTD)?
   A. Chemotherapy, with the regimen chosen based on prognostic factors
   B. Adjunctive pelvic radiation
   C. Avoiding future pregnancies
   D. Hysterectomy when childbearing is completed
   E. βhCG level every month after any future pregnancies

**Answers** • 1-B 2-C 3-E 4-D 5-A

## COMMENT

**Diagnosis of molar pregnancy** • Vaginal bleeding is the most common presenting complaint in molar pregnancies. Distinguishing between a molar pregnancy and an evolving abortion cannot be made with the information given, though a mole is suggested by the recurrence of nausea (caused by the high βhCG), increased uterine size, and elevated βhCG (the average maximum βhCG is 100,000 mIU/mL). A "snowstorm" appearance on ultrasound is pathognomonic for a complete mole. The diagnosis can also be made on a pathologic specimen after dilation and curettage, but an ultrasound should be done first. Disseminated intravascular coagulopathy (with elevated PT/PTT) can occur, but it is not diagnostic. A CT is not diagnostic. The CA125 test is more useful in epithelial ovarian cancers.

**Genetics of molar pregnancies** • There are two classes of moles: complete and incomplete. Complete moles usually present in the second trimester and are more often diagnosed on ultrasound than partial moles. A complete mole results from release of an ovum with no genetic material, which is then either fertilized by a sperm that duplicates itself or is fertilized by two sperm (46, XX represents 90% of cases; 46, YY is not seen, probably secondary to early abortion). Partial moles result from fertilization of a normal ovum by two sperm; the most common genotype is 69, XXY. 45, XO is Turner's syndrome, the most common specific genotype causing spontaneous abortions.

**Characteristics of partial and complete moles** • Aside from the genetic makeup that defines partial and complete moles, the clinical scenario is often quite different. In partial moles, fetus tissue is present (remembered by virtue of both maternal and paternal chromosomes being present). Diagnosis of partial moles is often made later than a complete mole, usually by the gynecologist or pathologist after dilation and curettage for second trimester spontaneous abortion. The associated conditions of vomiting, preeclampsia, hyperthyroidism, and theca-lutein cysts are more common in complete moles, due to the higher associated levels of βhCG. Persistence after evacuation is much more common with the complete mole (20% versus 4%), but βhCG must be followed closely with both types.

**Management of molar pregnancies** • The mainstay of therapy for both types of moles is surgical evacuation by dilation and curettage or evacuation. Blood loss can be significant, so typed and cross-matched blood is necessary. A βhCG level is important both as a prognostic factor for recurrence (higher if >100,000 mIU/mL at initial diagnosis) and as a marker to show regression. Effective contraception should be employed because a new pregnancy will give elevated βhCG levels, giving the impression of recurrence. βhCG levels should be drawn every week until *three consecutive* negative levels (0–5 mIU/mL) are obtained, then drawn *monthly* for 6 months. An increase or plateau over two consecutive cycles constitutes persistent disease.

**Management of persistent GTD** • Chemotherapy alone is extremely effective in GTD. With no evidence of metastasis, single-agent methotrexate is given (15–25 mg IM daily for 5 days). If metastases are present, treatment depends on prognostic factors, and may range from single-agent methotrexate to hysterectomy and three-agent chemotherapy. Poor prognostic factors include βhCG greater than 40,000 at the time of plateau; more than 4 months of disease; presence of brain or liver (not lung) metastases; failed prior chemotherapy; or GTD developed after term pregnancy. The incidence of a molar pregnancy with later pregnancies is just 1%. The next pregnancy should be closely monitored with early ultrasound, frequent visits, careful examination of any pathologic specimens, and assurance that βhCG levels return to normal after any pregnancy is completed. If no evidence of recurrence exists, a hysterectomy after completed childbearing is not necessary.

## CASE PRESENTATION

A 19-year-old woman presents to your office with the concern of not beginning her menstrual cycle. She has had no evidence of vaginal bleeding and is worried. She states all of her friends have gone through menarche. Her mother told her she is just a "late bloomer" and that her menses will come in time. She has no significant past medical history. She weighs 140 pounds and is 4 feet 11 inches tall. Her vitals are all within normal parameters. Exam reveals breast bud development. Normal external female genitalia are noted. She has a small uterus, which is mobile, anteverted and nontender. No adnexal masses are appreciated.

1. The normal progression of puberty is:
   A. Menarche, adrenarche, thelarche
   B. Adrenarche, menarche, thelarche
   C. Thelarche, menarche, adrenarche
   D. Thelarche, adrenarche, menarche
2. Which of the following laboratory values would be most helpful in establishing your diagnosis?
   A. Thyroid-stimulating hormone
   B. Prolactin
   C. Follicle-stimulating hormone
   D. Gonadotropin-releasing hormone
3. The lab value drawn returns with a value of 60. The most likely diagnosis is:
   A. Turner's syndrome
   B. Swyer's syndrome
   C. Rokitansky-Küster-Hauser syndrome
   D. 17-hydroxylase deficiency
4. If the lab value that was drawn returned with a value of 5, the only helpful step would be to order:
   A. CT of the pelvis
   B. CT of the head
   C. Ultrasound of the thyroid
   D. Ultrasound of the pelvis

## COMMENT

**Stages of pubertal development** • A series of physical changes due to the pubertal increase in androgen and estrogen occur prior to the onset of menses. A system referred to as Tanner stages I to V describes the five physical stages of breast and pubic hair development. The first physical sign usually associated with puberty is the beginning of breast development, known as *thelarche*. Thelarche stages progress from breast bud formation to a contoured breast with areola. Onset of thelarche is approximately 10 years of age. Thelarche is followed by *adrenarche,* the presence of axillary or pubic hair. Adrenarche typically occurs by age 12 but may precede thelarche in approximately 20% of children. The onset of menstrual periods, *menarche,* is the final stage of pubertal development. The average age of menarche in the United States is approximately 13 years. The diagnosis of primary amenorrhea is made when menarche has not occurred by age 16. The patient in this scenario should raise concern because there has been no breast development and no menarche by age 19. This should not be attributed to "a late bloomer" and deserves further workup.

**Laboratory tests** • Primary amenorrhea with physical findings of a normal uterus and no breast development can be divided into two distinct categories. These categories include *hypergonadotropic* hypogonadism and *hypogonadotropic* hypogonadism. Hypergonadotropic hypogonadism is caused by gonadal dysgenesis or gonadal failure. Because these patients have nonfunctioning ovaries and no estrogen production, the negative feedback of the hypothalamic pituitary ovarian axis results in an elevated follicle-stimulating hormone level. This is typically in the menopausal range, greater than 40 mIU/mL. Etiologies of hypergonadotropic hypogonadism include Turner's syndrome (45, XO), mosaicism, pure gonadal dysgenesis, and 17-hydroxylase deficiency.

**Genetic etiologies** • With a follicle-stimulating hormone level of 60 mIU/mL, this patient has the diagnosis of hypergonadotropic hypogonadism. The most common cause is Turner's syndrome (45, XO). Two X chromosomes are necessary for ovarian development. Turner's syndrome patients often develop fibrous bands of tissue called go nadal streaks. Due to decreased estrogen levels, breast development does not occur. Other characteristics of a patient with Turner's syndrome include short stature, short fourth metacarpal, webbed neck, and coarctation of the aorta. Although Swyer's syndrome (pure gonadal dysgenesis) and 17-hydroxylase enzyme deficiency are etiologies of hypergonadotropic hypogonadism, they are much more rare. Rokitansky-Küster-Hauser syndrome is Müllerian agenesis. This would not be a possible etiology of this patient because she has a normal pelvic exam.

**Hypothalamic and pituitary etiologies** • Hypogonadotropic hypogonadism is due to a hypothalamic or pituitary etiology resulting in decreased levels of follicle-stimulating hormone. Without adequate stimulation from follicle-stimulating hormone, the ovary is unable to secrete estrogen. Etiologies often include hypothalamic or pituitary congenital anatomical defects or a neoplasm such as a craniopharyngioma. Rare causes have been attributed to encephalitis and isolated neurotransmitter defects. Of the options listed, a CT of the head would be the most beneficial.

**Answers** • 1-D 2-C 3-A 4-B

## CASE PRESENTATION

A 34-year-old woman presents to your office with a 2-week history of a small ulceration on the left labia majora. She states it is nontender, and appears to be healing on its own. She is sexually active and does not use condoms. Her history is positive for *Chlamydia trachomatis* 2 years ago. She denies vaginal discharge or itching. Upon examination of the vulva you note a single ulceration, nontender to touch, with rolled edges. No other findings are noted.

1. You are most suspicious of:
   A. Herpes simplex virus (HSV) 2
   B. Chancroid
   C. Lichen sclerosis
   D. Syphilis
   E. None of the above
2. If this condition is not treated appropriately the next significant finding most likely will be:
   A. Maculopapular rash
   B. Neurological degeneration
   C. Continued thickening of labia majora
   D. Herpes simplex type 1
   E. None of the above
3. The most beneficial treatment for this condition is:
   A. Benzathine penicillin G IM
   B. Ceftriaxone 250 mg IM
   C. Clobetasol propionate ointment
   D. Oral acyclovir 200 mg 5 times daily for 7 days
   E. None of the above
4. Which of the following is the most appropriate test to diagnose the condition?
   A. Biopsy of the suspicious area
   B. HSV culture
   C. Fluorescent treponemal antibody absorption
   D. Culture for *Haemophilus ducreyi*
   E. None of the above

## COMMENT

**Vulvar ulcerations** • A *painless* indurated ulceration with rolled, smooth edges found on the vulva should immediately raise suspicion for primary syphilis. Herpes simplex type 2 is usually characterized by an outbreak of multiple, *painful* vesicular lesions. Herpes ulcers are typically superficial and inflamed. Because herpes may have multiple recurrences, a patient may give a history of similar findings. Chancroid presents as a painful single ulceration with irregular margins found deep within the vulva. Painful lymphadenopathy often accompanies chancroid. Lichen sclerosis would be very low on the differential diagnosis because this is considered a vulvar dystrophy, which is often seen in postmenopausal women. Lichen sclerosis is a benign condition of the vulva characterized by thinning of the epithelium leading to atrophic changes or agglutination of the labia. The vulvar skin is characterized by a white paperlike appearance. Patients often present with complaints of vulvar burning and itching.

**Stages of syphilis** • Primary syphilis is characterized by a painless vulvar ulceration referred to as a *chancre*. The chancre develops at the site of entry of the spirochete. A primary chancre typically develops 3 weeks after inoculation and usually heals without treatment within 2 to 6 weeks. If untreated, hematogenous dissemination occurs, leading to systemic disease—secondary syphilis. The characteristic finding associated with secondary syphilis is a red maculopapular rash, usually on the palms of hands and soles of feet. Secondary syphilis develops between 6 weeks and 6 months after the primary chancre has appeared. Tertiary syphilis may lead to degenerating effects on the nervous, musculoskeletal, and cardiovascular systems. Tertiary syphilis develops in greater than 30% of patients not treated during the primary, secondary, or latent stages.

**Treatment of syphilis** • The treatment of choice for primary, secondary, or early latent syphilis (syphilis of less than 1 year's duration) is a single dose of intramuscular 2.4 million units of benzathine penicillin G. Late latent syphilis (syphilis of more than 1 year's duration) is treated with three doses of 2.4 million units of benzathine penicillin G intramuscularly once a week for 3 consecutive weeks. The treatment for neurosyphilis is IV aqueous crystalline penicillin G for 14 days. Acyclovir is a treatment option for herpes simplex virus. Clobetasol propionate is a steroid cream used for abatement of lichen sclerosis. Ceftriaxone, a third-generation cephalosporin antibiotic, is usually first-line therapy for *Neisseria gonorrhoeae*. Antibiotic options for syphilis treatment in the penicillin-allergic patient include doxycycline, tetracycline, and erythromycin.

**Diagnostic tests** • Syphilis is caused by the spirochete *Treponema pallidum*. Spirochetes may be detected by dark-field microscopy from a smear of the ulceration. Because dark-field microscopy may be unavailable, two categories of serologic tests have been developed to identify syphilis. These include the nonspecific, nontreponemal tests and the specific, antitreponemal antibody tests. The nontreponemal tests used more for screening purposes are the VDRL (Venereal Disease Research Laboratories) test and the RPR (rapid plasma reagin) test. If a screening test is positive, it may be confirmed with the use of the FTA-ABS (fluorescent-labeled *Treponema* antibody absorption) or MHA-TP (microhemagglutination assay for antibodies to *Treponema pallidum*) antitreponemal antibody tests. Herpes simplex virus and chancroid, due to *Haemophilus ducreyi*, may both be detected by culture. Biopsy of the lesion would not be beneficial.

**Answers** • 1-D 2-A 3-A 4-C

## CASE PRESENTATION

A 55-year-old woman presents to the emergency room complaining of vaginal bleeding for a week. This is the first bleeding she has had in 7 years. She is using about two to three pads per day, and also reports a foul vaginal odor. Review of systems is negative. She is otherwise healthy, but smokes a pack of cigarettes a day. Her gynecologic history is significant for "abnormal" Pap smears in her 30s, which did not require treatment. She has not had a Pap smear in 10 years. Her pelvic exam is significant for a large cervix with an irregular, friable area at 12 o'clock. It begins bleeding vigorously when touched with the speculum, but is controlled with pressure applied with large cotton-tipped swabs.

1. This woman's greatest risk factor for having cervical cancer is:
   A. The symptom of post-menopausal bleeding
   B. Tobacco use
   C. 10 years since her last Pap smear
   D. History of abnormal Pap smear
   E. Age
2. The cervical lesion is biopsied in the emergency room. It returns showing squamous cell carcinoma. Which of the following cannot be used to stage the malignancy?
   A. Cervical biopsy specimen
   B. Suggestion of lymph adenopathy on a CT scan
   C. Intravenous pyelography
   D. Exam under anesthesia with cystoscopy and proctoscopy
   E. Chest radiograph
3. Exam under anesthesia is performed. A bulky (>5 cm) cervix is noted, and cystoscopy and proctoscopy are negative. The chest x-ray is negative. You assign a stage of IB2 cervical squamous cancer. Of the following, the best treatment for this patient is:
   A. Cold-knife conization
   B. Simple hysterectomy with bilateral salpingo-oophorectomy
   C. Simple hysterectomy with bilateral salpingo-oophorectomy and lymph node sampling
   D. Radical hysterectomy
   E. External beam radiation
4. A radical hysterectomy is performed, and the pathology report indicates bilateral lymph node involvement. Her stage is now:
   A. IB2
   B. IIA
   C. IIB
   D. IIIC
   E. IV

## COMMENT

**Risk factors for cervical cancer** • Cervical cancer is rare in women who obtain regular Pap smears and appropriate treatment. In fact, Pap smear screening is so effective that now the greatest risk factor for developing cervical cancer is failure to have appropriate screening. Although the other factors listed are associated with increased risk, they are not as high as failure to receive Pap smear screening.

**Staging of cervical cancer** • Unlike most cancers, which are surgically staged, cervical cancer is clinically staged. This means the designated stage is based on clinical findings of exam and lab tests, not the pathology specimen. Tests that can be used in staging include colposcopy, physical exam under anesthesia, cystoscopy and proctoscopy to evaluate bladder and rectum invasion, barium enema, chest x-ray to evaluate pulmonary metastasis, and intravenous pyelogram (IVP) to evaluate for hydronephrosis. The purpose of clinical staging is so that epidemiologic patterns can be evaluated consistently between different institutions, as well as between developed and underdeveloped countries, which may not have the resources to perform other than the above tests. This method of staging is being reconsidered. Patient management can be altered by results of other tests, such as a CT scan suggesting lymph node involvement, but the stage assigned remains clinical.

**Treatment of cervical cancer** • Stage I cervical cancers are those confined to the cervix only. For stage I and IIA lesions (involving a small portion of the vagina but not the parametrial tissue), radical hysterectomy and radiation therapy are equally curative. The therapy of choice depends on which risks are more acceptable to the patient. For relatively young patients who are at low risk of complications from surgery, radical hysterectomy is preferred. This avoids the long-term complications of radiation therapy that last a lifetime, such as radiation enteritis and fistula formation (once radiated, always radiated). For older patients and those at high surgical risk, such as significant cardiovascular or pulmonary disease, radiation therapy may provide the more favorable risk/benefit profile.

A simple hysterectomy does not remove the parametrial tissue (uterosacral, cardinal, and broad ligaments) necessary to provide maximal chance of cure from excision. A cold-knife conization is appropriate in microinvasive cancers of the cervix.

**Staging recurrent or progressing cervical cancer** • Because cervical cancer is clinically staged, it does not change based on operative or pathologic findings. Even if patients present with metastatic recurrence years later, the original clinical stage assigned is kept.

**Answers** • 1-C 2-B 3-D 4-A

# • Index

## D



## E



## F



## G

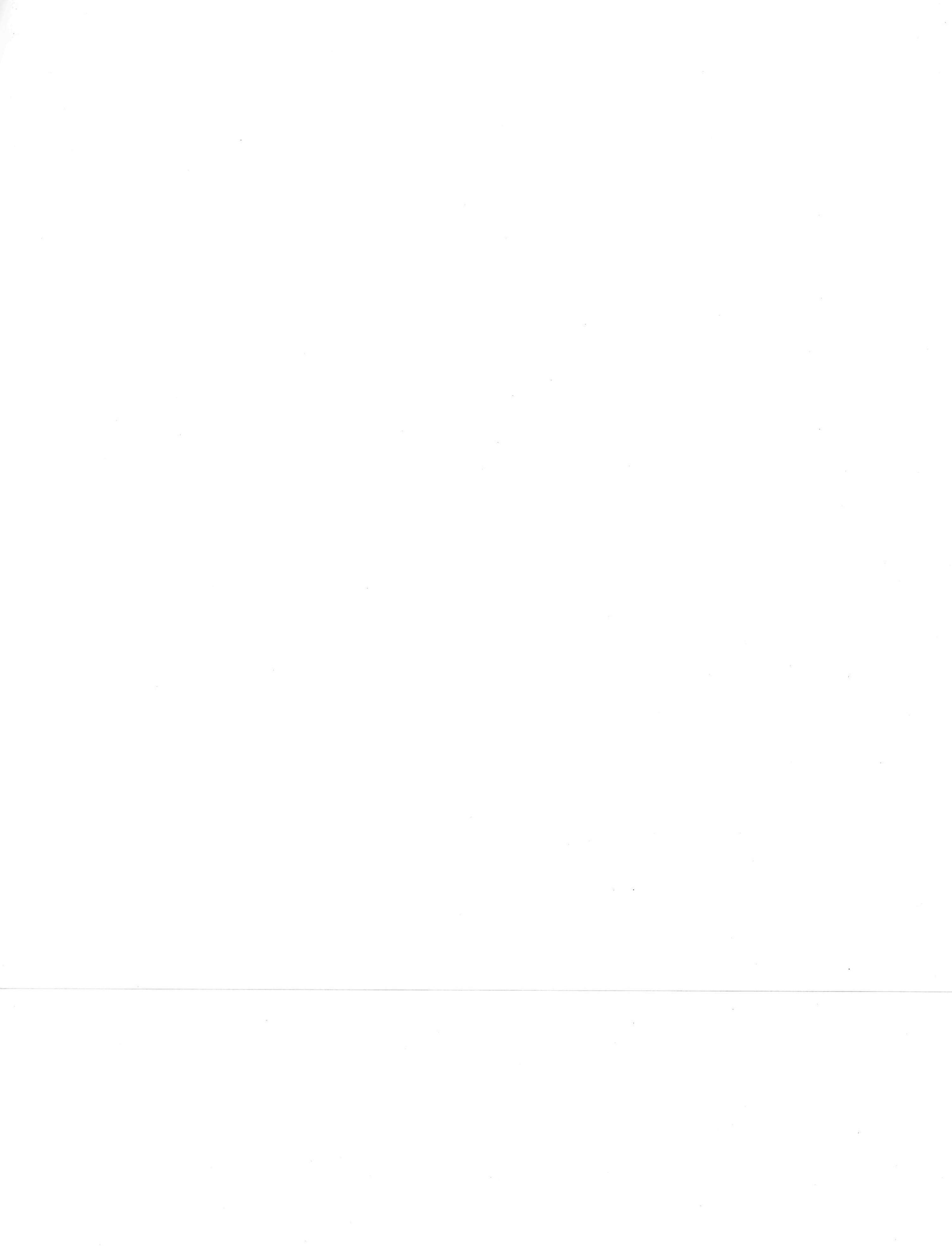